PARKINSONIAN
Democracy

A LEGAL FICTION ADVOCATING DIET AND
EXERCISE FOR PARKINSON'S

JERRY HURTUBISE, J.D.

PARKINSONIAN DEMOCRACY

A LEGAL FICTION

JERRY HURTUBISE, J.D.

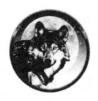

First Edition

ISBN: 978-1-947782-15-0

Publisher info: Winterwolf Press

Website: WinterwolfPress.com

Cover art and Cover design by Jose M. Bethencourt

Interior design by Christine Contini

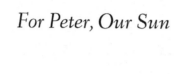

For Peter, Our Sun

CONTENTS

PREFACE

We learn from an early age that we are endowed by our Creator with certain inalienable rights such as life, liberty, and the pursuit of happiness, but what never seems to get equal attention is that in order to maximize the benefits of these lofty ideals, we each have also been given the freedom to gravitate toward and activate the rational part of our brain designed for the purpose of making the best decisions.

At this stage of our evolution, it seems to have become part of the human condition for many of us to opt out of using the smartest part of our brain (the frontal lobe) to address life-changing issues and, instead, choose to do much of our thinking from other, less enlightened parts of the brain, which may simply be fertile breeding grounds for fear, prejudice, and unhealthy addictions.

I first became aware of the phenomenon of what is referred to as competing areas of the brain while litigating head trauma cases, where it became clear that when a person suffered a devastating injury to the frontal lobe, it did not mean he or she stopped thinking, but rather that it often meant he or she would end up having to process thought from other, less rational parts of the brain designed for other purposes.

The good news for most of us who have been diagnosed with Parkinson's disease is we still have the choice of taking full advantage of using our prefrontal cortex to fully assess the advantages of moving toward a medical model that incorporates the critical role, no, really, the critical role diet and exercise play in the remedial equation and, as I will argue, the challenges of relying solely upon prescription medications as an exclusive remedy.

In order to achieve all the benefits of taking what for some may be seen as the path of *most* resistance, it will be necessary to unpack some of what science has discovered about the human brain over the last century, not the least of which is the notion that decision making regarding important matters such as how to domesticate a progressive brain disease is best understood from the vantage point of the rational part of the brain.

Assume for the sake of argument that this is true, then it also stands to reason that whether we become healthy or

unhealthy, or, for that matter, love or hate, evolve or de-
volve, have character or simply become characters, be
prophets or profiteers, will in large part depend on
which particular competing area of the brain we choose
to end up using.

If, for example, we condition ourselves—or, probably
more likely, allow ourselves to be conditioned—to generate most of our thoughts from our anger (fight) or fear
(flight) centers (amygdala), rather than from the part of
the brain intended for processing rational thought (the
prefrontal cortex) or from the part intended to appreciate the consequences of behavior (the orbitofrontal
cortex), it should come as no surprise that where we
choose to process thought will greatly influence the
choices we make.

Indeed, the evidence will show it is critical from the get-
go to streamline an unencumbered pathway to the rational brain without being bogged down by such things
as anger or guilt.

The evidence, then, to be offered in the following legal
fiction, timely filed in the United States District Court
of Public Opinion, will show that depending upon
which competing area of the brain we gravitate to activate, it may very well determine how we react to our
being diagnosed with Parkinson's disease, and, thus, decisions yet to be made may very well affect the quality of

our lives and, more importantly, the quality of the lives of those whom we love.

To that end, it is strongly advised that exclusive neurological jurisdiction in all manners in which thought is processed should be discharged at or near the prefrontal cortex, what will become known as the only highly evolved part of the brain having the aptitude and judicial temperament necessary to solve any problem, especially if fear, prejudice, or an unhealthy addiction, with malice aforethought, attempts to control the narrative.

If the following experiment is allowed to run its course, we, more likely than not, will, in the end, not only be able to see more clearly how the aforementioned obstacles prevent us from achieving our optimal health physically, but, also, how these impetuous suspects conspire to prevent us from achieving our optimal mental and spiritual health as well.

With that in mind, let us all rise to the occasion.

Parkinsonians,
          Plaintiffs,   Case No. 01-10-1953

                                      CLASS ACTION
    v.

A Traditional Medical Paradigm,
          Defendants

TO: ALL WHO SUFFER OR WILL SUFFER A PROGRESSIVE BRAIN DISEASE

Introduction
Honorable Abraham Solomon

"Ladies and Gentlemen of the jury, my name is Judge Abraham Solomon and I have been appointed to preside over the matter of *Parkinsonians vs. A Traditional Medical Paradigm*, Case Number 01-10-1953, which has been duly filed in a timely manner in the United States District Court of Public Opinion, Northern District of California.

"Counsel for the Plaintiffs is Christian Cultura, who has agreed to represent *Parkinsonians*, described as a class of citizens all of whom have been diagnosed with a progressive brain disease referred to as Parkinson's and who have agreed to listen to evidence without passion or prejudice regarding the modern trend of using diet and exercise as a way of slowing down the progression of their disease in conjunction with the use of prescription medications.

"The Defendant, *A Traditional Medical Paradigm*, represented by Big Farma John, choosing not to make a formal appearance, has, nonetheless, given the Court permission to argue that throughout most of its history, prescription medications have been the exclusive remedy for treating Parkinson's disease and the modern trend is setting a very dangerous precedent by suggesting the use of diet and exercise can be used on the same par with prescription medications as a way of dealing with this dreaded illness.

"Mr. Cultura, intends to respond by showing medications should no longer be perceived as an exclusive remedy for those who suffer from Parkinson's, but, instead, by a preponderance of the evidence, intends to prove that the critical way in which we cope with Parkinson's disease, can be likened to a three legged stool; one leg representing diet, another exercise and a third being medical treatment.

"In helping to prove his case, Counsel requests at the outset of the proceedings, the Court make a special finding which emphasizes how important it is for those who review the evidence in this action to do so only from the more enlightened areas of the brain which have evolved down through time for purposes having to do with rational thinking and problem solving.

Otherwise, he is concerned some of those whom he represents may be unable to act in their own best interest, especially if they allow themselves to be overcome by fear, prejudice or addiction, which are percepts common to other areas of the brain which have evolved for survival purposes having little to do with executive decision making.

"What this court finds of some interest, is that Mr. Cultura feels to which area of the brain we choose to gravitate to activate will not only show how we end up acting upon critical evidence when deciding how diet and exercise fits into the equation of how we treat a progressive brain disease, but also, as a collateral matter, he intends to show the remarkable similarity of how we use the same mental gymnastics when deciding what kind of world in which we want to live.

"With regards to this particular collateral issue, he is inclined to think there may be some larger social benefit yet to be discovered in plain view, this court is willing to give Counsel wide latitude to present any evidence he feels is necessary to prove his theory that competing areas of the brain has even wider ramifications on our culture than simply as to how we might choose to treat a pesky brain disease.

"Big Farma John, on the other hand, in addition to rebuking any notion suggesting the Parkinson's population needs anything beyond prescription medications to treat the disease, wants it stated for the record that Counsel's theory of competing areas of the brain is totally irrelevant in these proceedings for any purpose whatsoever, and, besides, Counsel is not competent to offer any opinions related to brain chemistry because he lacks the credentials on the subject.

"Mr. Cultura, as an aside, begs the Court's indulgence to state for the record, if diet and aerobic exercise is used as a way of aiding in the treatment of Parkinson's disease, said decision should only be made with the close <u>supervision, care and permission</u> of a medical doctor.

"And, also, all members of the Class and their genetically vulnerable progeny, should be warned that since the causes of Parkinson's disease vary greatly from individual to individual, Mr. Cultura offers no guarantees as to the effectiveness and/or safety of his or any aerobic program or dietary suggestions.

"Mr. Cultura openly admits the preceding disclaimer is shamelessly self-serving, but insists it be made part of the record, nonetheless, as a legal reflex thing.

"When attempting to prove his case, he also gives fair warning, he will attempt to use humor and creative imagery such as referring to DNA as Distant Nomadic Ancestors.

"In that vein, Counsel boldly asserts his method of using intense aerobic therapy, as a way of coping with Parkinson's disease, by attempting to jump start and restore the electro-chemical life left in his remaining brain cells, can be likened to how he recharges the dying cells in a car battery.

"The difference being, rather than going through the labor intensive process of hooking little jumper cables to billions and billions of tiny brain cells each day, he, instead, attempts to induce an aerobic high on an elliptical machine thereby flooding oxygen into his brain to get a similar electrical charge.

"*A Traditional Medical Paradigm*, whose strategy will be not to give this matter 'more attention than it deserves', again, wants the record to reflect relying upon diet and exercise as primary forms of treatment, on equal footing with prescription medications, 'is frivolous and dangerous to the common good' and falls remarkably short of any traditional standards, historic accepted customs or practices or tested guidelines in the medical community.

"And it also warns the Court of Public Opinion to be very wary of Christian Cultura, arguing he will stop at nothing, including his feeble attempt at humor used solely as a distraction to trick the hearts and minds of a vulnerable population.

"To that end, Big Farma John has petitioned the Court to read into the record a portion of an *amicus* (friend of the court) brief, written by the Honorable Bobby Jingoism from the great state of Alabama, where the judge ends a nearly one hundred page scathing attack on the character of Christian Cultura, by concluding, 'Look only to the letter of the law and not to Mr. Cultura's self-serving and hauntingly absurd spirit of the law, where it has been shown on many occasion he will stop at nothing to use his devilish charm as a scoundrel might to lure a blind alley cat off a shrimp boat.'

"Finally, Ladies and Gentlemen, as a bookkeeping matter, it should be noted for the record my opening comments were reviewed and approved by all parties and the record should further reflect, all parties have stipulated to waive strict compliance with the Federal Rules of Evidence for the sake of judicial economy.

"The Court now awaits to hear Mr. Cultura's opening statement."

CHAPTER 1
PARK IN THE SUN

"MAY it please the Court and all those who are here present, most especially esteemed members of the Court of Public Opinion.

"My name is Christian Cultura, and I represent a wide range of people whose paths would not have crossed with mine save for our having been diagnosed at different stages of our lives with any number of progressive brain diseases, most specifically, Parkinson's disease.

"These proceedings will begin as they will end, with the notion that we each have within our control the freedom to premeditate and deliberate on how to cause chemical reactions in our brain that are so electrically charged that they result in keeping brain cells alive so we might continue to be clear thinkers and a body in motion for as long as we all shall live.

"As suggested by the Court, and for good reason, all evidence presented in these proceedings should be weighed from the only part of the brain capable of entertaining rational thought.

"Processing thought in the frontal lobe is important for many reasons, not the least of which is that it greatly reduces the risk that any progress we make will be hijacked by fear, passion, or prejudice, which are thought based emotions harvested in other parts of the brain that have evolved for reasons other than critical thinking and problem solving.

"To bring clarity and to help illustrate this point, as His Honor has eluded, evidence will be presented to show what happens in a much larger social context when these particular manifestations of thought, i.e., fear, passion, and prejudice, are allowed to dominate the way we think, thus being left unchecked by the more evolved and enlightened part of the brain capable of rational thought.

"I first became aware of this phenomenon while litigating closed head injuries, when my expert witnesses would make a very compelling argument that just because a person suffered a trauma to his or her brain causing permanent damage to their prefrontal cortex, the region involved in higher level cognition, other, less rational, competing areas of the brain would attempt to fill the void, almost always with undesirable consequences.

"So there is no confusion about how important it is for the prefrontal cortex to win the rivalry between competing areas of the brain; it bears repeating. Our case will include illustrations intended to dramatize the unintended consequences of how history tends to keep repeating itself when we, collectively, insist on processing thought and acting upon it from parts of the brain more reptilian in nature and designed for other, more immediate survival purposes."

"COUNSEL, can you be clearer by explaining to the court what all this has to do with the care and treatment of Parkinson's disease?"

"YOUR HONOR, when a person is first diagnosed with a progressive brain disease, as in the case of Parkinson's, there is a good chance the person will react by moving toward either becoming paralyzed with fear or having prejudice against being advised on issues related to diet and exercise, or may even find ephemeral consolation in an unhealthy addiction, all reactions easy to understand after having been given some pretty shocking news.

"By highlighting these particular problems (fear, prejudice, and addiction) in a larger social context and by showing the destruction they are each capable of doing if allowed to fester, it will help to illustrate how important it is for those of us who have been diagnosed with Parkinson's to understand why it is important to resolve these issues before they are allowed to get out of control and somehow end up causing much in the way of unnecessary harm to our mind and body."

"PLEASE CONTINUE, COUNSEL."

"SO YOUR HONOR, I intend, therefore, to prove by using truth based rational thought, processed at or near the frontal lobe, that our best hope for gaining a deeper appreciation of how to best cope with Parkinson's disease is done by proving to the rational brain how diet and exercise can work in harmony with medications being recommended by a movement disorder specialist."

"CAN you provide us with an example, Counsel?"

"WHY YES, it will become clear that every time our intent is to induce an aerobic high, the evidence will show and the unencumbered rational brain will understand, we are effectively responsible for the electrical stimulation of brain cells in the part of the basal ganglia, the substantia nigra, the degeneration of which causes Parkinson's, and that relevant part, along with other motor parts of the brain, get 'tricked' into thinking all this out of the ordinary motor movement likely means a survival issue is afoot, or more likely 'a-claw,' causing neurons to operate at their full potential to avert what our prehistoric ancestors rightly perceived as an existential threat. (Reference, Paul E. Hurtubise, PhD, Ohio State University (1976); former Director of Immunology Laboratory, Professor and Emeritus Professor of Pathology, University of Cincinnati College of Medicine, 1976-2017).

"The evidence, then, will show an unencumbered rational brain is more likely to understand that orchestrating a runner's high may be the key to unlocking and, thus, stimulating billions and billions of movement-friendly postsynaptic receptors, i.e., the antennas of the brain cells, which have been, evolutionarily speaking, one of the reasons we were able to have survived through some pretty dicey eras."

"CAN YOU EXPLAIN, Counsel, how this so-called 'unlocking' of postsynaptic receptors works?"

. . .

"WE WILL GET MORE into how brain cells function as the evidence is presented, your Honor, but for now, using a helpful analogy shared with me by a brilliant chemist, neurons can be likened to billions and billions of microscopic latchkey kids (brain cells), who have been sharpening their skills to adapt over time by chiseling their keys (neurotransmitters) to be able to fit perfectly into compatible locks (postsynaptic receptors) of other latchkey kids (brain cells) with the evolutionary intent of passing along different types of information depending on what part of the brain is being stimulated. (Reference, Robert Hurtubise, PhD, Ohio University (1969); Professor and former Chair, Department of Chemistry, University of Wyoming, 1974-2008).

"So, your Honor, I suppose the issue before the court is whether it is better for someone learning to adapt to the challenges of Parkinson's disease 'to be (a body at rest) or not to be (a body at rest), that is the question, and if one chooses the latter, whether a body in motion truly does stay in motion.' (Crossover Citation, Sir Isaac Newton (1643-1727) and William Shakespeare, (1561-1616)."

. . .

"COUNSEL, before you go off on a tangent, share with the court your early experience with Parkinson's disease."

"WELL, your Honor, after being diagnosed, I initially fell prey to allowing Parkinson's panic to control my thoughts from a more primitive part of my brain rather than thinking rationally from my frontal lobe.

"Indeed, it wasn't until I attended a Parkinson's symposium in a plush hotel in downtown San Francisco that a fog tightly clinging to the more primordial part of my brain would be lifted.

"As I sat fidgeting under the warm glow of crystal chandeliers, probably used more often to refract light for happier events like wedding receptions and bar mitzvah parties, my rational thought was no match for my fear until the keynote speaker informed us, 'Parkinson's is a progressive brain disease which will take from each of you, one thing at a time, (longer than necessary pregnant pause), one by one, until, in the end, there is nothing left for it to take.'

"It seems as though being sentenced to a death by a million Parkinson paper cuts was all it took for me to transition from being a person incarcerated in a cell of his fear center (the amygdala) to someone moving toward a more reasonable way of adapting to his fate.

"So, with all due respect, your Honor, the speaker's sweeping generalization, foreboding the inevitable outcome for all who had Parkinson's disease, seemed to be objectionable on many grounds, including that it assumes facts that are not in evidence."

"EXPLAIN, COUNSEL!"

"WELL, your Honor, the assumption that a person is going to sit idly by and let things be permitted to be taken away 'one by one' is in itself not based on any clear and convincing evidence.

"Even with that said, I must admit, your Honor, that his words did have a chilling effect on me, especially since body parts already affected by the disease, to which I had grown quite attached, like my arms and legs, were on a course to prove his theory correct."

"ARE you referring to your own symptoms, Counsel, and if you are, can you name a few?"

. . .

"YES, your Honor, first there was a tremor in my right hand, which I referred to as Elvis because in it there was 'a whole lotta shakin' goin' on.'

"Second, a weakening voice is not considered a bad thing by those distrustful of trial lawyers.

"Third, the expression of my appearing sad, much the way Timmy must have felt when Lassie ran away, made him look 'melon-collie.'

"And, fourth, illustrative of the preceding symptom, I seem to be suffering from an inability to refrain from spewing out offensive humor that happens to pop into my head, which, by the way, is a symptom of the disease not yet recognized by any self-respecting health care professional."

"THANK YOU, Counsel, for alerting the Court of your last symptom. It does indeed sound particularly offensive."

"YOUR HONOR, for the record, I will say if my bad jokes become problematic in these proceedings, I would understand it if the Court found it necessary to issue a 'gag' order."

. . .

"IF SUCH SOPHOMORIC ANTICS ARE, indeed, displayed in open court, I will decide at that time how to deal with them."

"THANK YOU, YOUR HONOR."

"LET'S now get back to the subject at hand, Counsel."

"YES, your honor, of course. To defend the keynote speaker, I was going to say that his forthrightness did dispel any hope I had that Parkinson's disease could be cured in the near future, and that, in a sense, he was admitting that medication alone as a means of treating the disease was not a formula for keeping brain cells alive, which seems to be the main problem.

"So even though he found the weakest link in my daisy chain of denial, the guest speaker did set in motion the incentive I would need to seek and find the best way for me to treat my Parkinson's disease, and if I had any measure of success, I could share it with others similarly situated."

. . .

"COUNSEL, does that conclude your opening statement?"

"YES, your Honor, but before I begin my case-in-chief, I am sensing there is someone amongst us who recently has been diagnosed with Parkinson's disease and who needs to hear the words, 'All shall be well, and all manner of things shall be well.'" (Citation, Julian of Norwich, Christian mystic, 1352-1416).

"AND WHY DO you feel this is important, Counsel?"

"WELL, your Honor, it may help that person understand he or she will never walk alone.

"With that said, I would also like to say to anyone, the person, maybe, who is sad and may be having a dark night of the soul after learning of the diagnosis, that a grief reaction is normal, but should be viewed in the context of as having a beginning and an end and once it slowly fades into the next phase of life, a plethora of hope not only awaits, but also a community of people with unimaginable inner beauty."

CHAPTER 2
GUNK SCIENCE

"YOUR HONOR, I would like to begin by saying the evidence will show how important it is for people diagnosed with Parkinson's disease to incorporate the proper diet and daily exercise into their world—a world in which, until recently, taking prescription drugs in doses commensurate with escalating symptoms was pretty much the only game in town.

"It should also be mentioned at the outset that, although these prescription medications can be quite effective at controlling symptoms, a small segment of the Parkinson's population stands the risk of suffering side effects that may be greater than the actual symptoms of the disease itself.

"Indeed, for whatever reason, their ungalvanized genes may not be coated with nearly enough armor to match the shock and awe of these chemical weapons, which makes getting the right prescription and seeing a movement disorder specialist all the more important."

"OKAY, Counsel, point is taken. How do you now wish to proceed?"

"SO, your Honor, in order to set the stage, I would like to begin by offering into evidence some vocabulary, which will be helpful because it will give us a better understanding of how the brain works, and this, in turn, will give us the context we need to know why it is so critically important to keep brain cells alive in order to slow down the progression of the disease to a snail's pace.

"First is the word *nucleus*, which, here, can be defined as a band of like-minded brain cells, the purpose or function of which will depend upon to which area of the brain they have evolved in order to pass along electrically charged signals from neuron to neuron or brain cell to brain cell.

"Using an analogy that may be helpful to some, a nucleus can be likened to a street gang made up of gang members (brain cells), who have evolved to a specific neighborhood in the brain because they (brain cells) share the same territorial function.

"And depending on which brain turf the gang (nucleus) has evolved, e.g., the motor cortex, this will be the overriding factor in determining which function is expected of gang members (brain cells).

"Everything works swimmingly so long as electrically signaled information is able to be communicated with like minded cells, some of which stay close to home (interneurons), while others are designed to project out beyond their nucleus of origin to other gangs (another nucleus).

"Before we get carried away, your Honor, with too much in the way of the gang imagery, which may to some suggest criminal intent, it should be of some comfort to the Court to know that even though these interconnected brain chain *gangs* are territorial, each gang (nucleus) has become remarkably democratic in the way it shares electrochemically charged information with other gangs, probably because their mutual survival is dependent upon sharing of information.

"In that vein, signaled *survival* information, then, from gang to gang, nucleus to nucleus, can also be visualized as free flowing information highways or neuropaths, the streamlining of which remains constant, at least until gang members (brain cells) become what I refer to as *gunked.*"

"GUNKED, COUNSEL?"

"YES, your Honor, *gang* members (brain cells), I believe, may die if they become congested with too much protein or filaments, which are normal in the right amounts but in excess can gum up or gunk up the inner workings of a brain cell.

"Gunk science, by analogy, is probably more easily understood in the context of how gunk clogs up heart valves when we suffer the unintended consequences of an arterial coronary traffic jam due, maybe, to way too many *gunkin' donuts* or, to be fair, any food that causes an excess amount of blockage, i.e., excess amounts of saturated fats or sugar laden processed foods.

"The contextual understanding of how the heart can die is enhanced even more when one can actually see, via a scan, how gunk blocks heart valves or, closer to home, plaque or bacteria gunk up arteries in the brain, causing an ischemic stroke.

"This 'seeing is believing' phenomenon is probably why cardiologists are way ahead of the curve when singing the praises of aerobic exercise as a way of helping heart valves remain a gunk free zone.

"In all fairness, your Honor, neurologists, with a growing number of exceptions, have not been as enthusiastic over the last century about singing the praises of aerobic movement, because it hasn't been until recently, with the advent of magnetic resonance imaging (MRI), that cellular voyeurism has even been able to suggest the part we unwittingly play in our own neuronal genocide.

"So, your Honor, gunk science can be best understood, microscopically, in the context of when brain cells suffer a fatality; their tiny death certificates might read, under cause of death, 'Got gunked.'"

"CAN you cite examples of where brain cells can suffer from gunking?"

"YES, your Honor, just a few examples of my theory of Gunk Science are:

1. Abnormal accumulations of clumps of a protein called *Lewy bodies* in brain cells in a part of the basal ganglia (substantia nigra) cause these little fellows to die, which, when this neuronal genocide gets out of control, can cause Parkinson's.

2. Excessive clumps of a protein called *amyloid* (Amy Lloyd) in brain cells of the hippocampus, which stores memory, are thought to be a cause of Alzheimer's Disease.

3. Too much of a protein called *tau*, twisting and turning into filaments, is thought to cause frontotemporal dementia.

4. Too many oligodendrocytes, support cells for neurons called glial cells, which help them to conduct electrical charges down the axon, are thought to cause brain tumors when in excess or multiple sclerosis (MS) when there are not enough. (Reference, *The Dementias*, National Institute of Neurological Disorders and Stroke, NIH Publication No. 13-2252, September 2013)."

"COUNSEL, help the Court understand how brain cells pass information between one another."

"OKAY, your Honor, the relative space between brain cells, over which chemically charged information passes, is called the *synapse*, thus bringing terms like *presynaptic terminals* (the launching pad on the sender cell) and *postsynaptic receptors* (the first stop on receiving information on the sendee cell).

"Chemical information, then, is carried across this synapse via neurotransmitters, and when the neuro-transmitters interact with receptors on the postsynaptic membrane, the signal or information continues on its journey.

"It is important to note some neurotransmitters are *excitatory* (e.g., acetylcholine, aspartate, noradrenalin, gluta-mate, and histamine) and some are *inhibitory* (e.g., gamma amino butyric acid, glycine, and serotonin).

"One neurotransmitter of particular importance to us, dopamine, because of its relationship to Parkinson's, is both excitatory and inhibitory, suggesting to me that even though both are dopamine, their respective neuro-transmitting key capacities must unlock different types of postsynaptic receptors.

"Again, with our earlier latchkey kid analogy in mind, the chemicals in the key (neurotransmitters) go over the synapse, and if the key fits, it unlocks the postsynaptic receptor on what is called a dendrite, which are often described as looking like tree branches, but considering all the electricity involved, would probably more accurately be thought of as a television antenna gone wild.

"The purpose of unlocking the next cell lock in the cell block is to open a portal, my word, through which a cavalcade of ions (charged atoms) go into a user friendly cell, past its cell body, and to a place called the axon hillock, where it is determined whether there is to be an *action potential*.

"Assuming the information has action potential or is, in fact, information worthy, it continues down a 'long' corridor, again, space being relative, called an *axon*, and although every synoptically charged event is measured in milliseconds, the more the axon is myelinated, again, by glial or support cells called oligodendrocytes, the faster the information travels. (Remember when myelin is somehow defective on the axon then multiple sclerosis can result.)

"Parenthetically—it is also important to know when the metabolic recipes of glucose breaking down in various ways, intended to create the energy the neuron needs–if any of this is somehow compromised, this can be yet another way in which brain cells run the risk of dying. (Reference, Daniel A. Friedman, BS, University of California, Davis (2014), PhD, Ecology and Evolution, Stanford University, 2019)

"It is also noteworthy—something which will be explored in more detail later—that there are good foods for the brain, which will determine how healthy a brain cell will become, and there are bad foods for a brain cell, which will determine how unhealthy a brain cell will become, putting it at greater risk of dying."

. . .

"IT IS SO NOTED, COUNSEL."

"YOUR HONOR, I would now like the Court to understand the word "information" as it relates to what is being passed between brain cells, the information of which will vary depending upon the particular part of the brain that is being activated."

"COUNSEL, PLEASE CONTINUE."

"SO, your Honor, the scientific miracle of how information is passed between brain cells at electrical speeds hard to fathom has been fine-tuning itself for millions of years and explains how we have been able to survive threats, predatory and otherwise.

"What is important to understand is that information passing between neurons is not just about passing knowledge or thoughts as we typically think about or define information."

"CAN you give the Court an example of what you mean, Counsel?"

. . .

"WELL, for example, if brain cells in the part of the brain called the limbic system are passing electrically charged information, that information probably has to do with memory, emotion, or learning (MEL), which is the way most of us typically think about how to define information.

"On the other hand, another part of the brain called the reticular formation, found in the brain stem, passes information from cell to cell having to do with things we take for granted like breathing, sleeping, and heart-beating.

"And what is most relevant for us to know, in light of these proceedings, is that brain cells in the primary motor cortex, premotor cortex, cerebellum (coordination), and extrapyramidal motor system communicate movement information.

"Since motor neurons are interdependent and interconnected, sharing vital movement information, it is easy to understand how, when brain cells start dying off relatively exponentially, thus no longer being able to pass movement information from cell to cell, a person having been diagnosed with Parkinson's might end up moving around like a couple of "wild and crazy guys." (Reference, *Saturday Night Live* bit, circa 1978, where "two wild and crazy guys," the Czech-born Festrunk brothers, Yortuk (Dan Aykroyd) and Georg (Steve Martin), are on the constant prowl for "American foxes")."

"SO WHAT YOU ARE SAYING, Counsel, is that when a particular motor program loses a threshold number of brain cells, it may no longer be able to coordinate movement, and the more brain cells lost, the more erratic movement can become."

"YES, your Honor, and, again, this happens in Parkinson's disease when a nucleus in the brain called the substantia nigra, found in the basal ganglia, loses more than half of its brain cells, and as a result, people may have a whole host of things that can go wrong, including having tremors, not being able to swing their arms back and forth when they walk, or even being found to lack coordination, i.e., "I'm not drunk, I have Parkinson's.""

"I GUESS you could say that by the time you are diagnosed with Parkinson's, your cup is half empty, Counsel."

. . .

"WITH DUE RESPECT, I would rather think of my substantia nigra cup as still being half full, and my challenge is figuring out how to prevent the loss of even more brain cells."

"IT'S time to move onto another subject, Counsel."

CHAPTER 3
THE SCENE OF THE CRIME

"HOW DO you wish to proceed, Counsel?"

"IF OUR NUMBER one objective is to figure out a way of keeping brain cells alive so we might be able to move as best we can, it might be helpful to become familiar with the areas not only inside a brain cell but also in regions surrounding them and even exploring areas further away from the neuron, which may be important as well."

"PLEASE CONTINUE, COUNSEL."

. . .

"SO, then, your Honor, if the Court is willing to accept the premise that a progressive brain disease like Parkinson's progresses because brain cells are dying at an alarming rate and thus are no longer able to do what they were intended to do, which is to pass along *movement* information, their untimely deaths, as suggested, may be caused by a constellation of different reasons.

"For example, the evidence will show that the health of a brain cell is greatly affected by the health of *astrocytes*."

"ASTRO SIGHTS, COUNSEL?"

"AN ASTROCYTE IS a star shaped support cell surrounding a neuron that has been evolutionarily charged to do some heavy duty neuronal parenting since they are designed to protect the brain cell to which they were assigned, from toxic waste, provide them with the nutrients we feed the brain, keep them insulated, and, more recently, have been thought to play an important role in memory and sleep, kind of like what parents do for their children.

"And, perhaps, since we know there are legions of these cellular patriarchs and matriarchs outside a neuron, your Honor, it may be worth discovering more about bad things that can happen outside the brain cell when something goes wrong with astrocytes, where, for example, they are no longer able to perform their duties and neurons are left to fend for themselves.

"Just saying, your Honor, going beyond the crime scene of the actual inside of the brain cell to look at who or what has access to or motive to kill a neuron, maybe free radicals, ties in well with research suggesting '...We need to rethink the way we look at brain metabolism. Understanding the precise and biological mechanisms of the brain is a critical first step in disease-based research. Any misconception about biological functions—such as <u>metabolism</u>—will ultimately impact how scientists form a hypothesis and analyze their findings. **If we are looking in the wrong place, we won't be able to find the right answers.**' (Citation, Maiken Nidergaard, M.D., D.M.Sc., Co-director, University of Rochester Center for Translational Neuro-Medicine, *Understanding How Nerve Cells in the Brain Produce Energy Required to Function*, News-Medical.net, 2015, Emphasis added).

"Your Honor, under the heading of possibly looking in the wrong place, there is emerging research that strongly suggests that other parts of our anatomy, other than just the brain, should be subpoenaed and brought in for questioning for suspicion of conspiring with malice aforethought to be a proximate cause of Parkinson's disease, i.e., the killing of brain cells.

"Indeed, there is, for example, mounting evidence of 'a major link between gut microbes and PD.' (Michael S. Okun, M.D., *Gut Bacteria and H.pylori*, Parkinson Report, National Parkinson Foundation, Spring, 2017)

"THE POINT OF THIS EXERCISE, your Honor, is that becoming aware that there may be a laundry list of reasons why brain cells are dying will later assist the Court in showing not only how the legal doctrine of proximate cause may be used to explain how a particular person may have been diagnosed with Parkinson's disease, but also might help in explaining how diet and exercise may just become superseding intervening events able to prevent a particular proximate cause from escalating beyond a point of no return."

"COUNSEL, why wait until later in these proceedings to explain the legal theory of proximate cause, which for our purposes can be defined as uncovering what are the substantial factor(s) that are most responsible for bringing about the disease?"

. . .

"YOUR HONOR, before connecting the dots, it is crucial we make sure no one is suffering from any fear, prejudice, or addiction that might taint his or her perception of the evidence, otherwise, all we will be doing is giving away ice in the wintertime."

"COUNSEL, again, I promised to give you wide latitude in your attempts to prove how fear, prejudice, or an addiction can threaten a person's ability to think rationally as it relates to health care, but I might ask if you can give the Court some guidance as to how you intend to do this."

"YOUR HONOR, I believe the best way to drive home my point as to how a misplaced fear, an unreliable prejudice, or an unhealthy addiction has the power to distort the truth presented in these proceedings is to put into evidence examples that show their destructive power in a way in which we can all relate.

"Indeed, to hammer home my point, I intend, for example, to show how when a society permits itself to manufacture fright with reckless abandon, runaway fear, manifesting itself into anger, would risk the culture being diagnosed with a personality disorder if it were judged by the same psychological standards as that of an individual."

"AGAIN, the Court is inclined to give you latitude, but I do expect you to get back on track by returning to the legal theory of proximate cause and how it can relate to Parkinson's disease."

"YOU HAVE my word that I will address that particular issue, your Honor, once it is understood how fear, prejudice and addictions can get in the way of a person being able to think rationally in circumstances having to do with a progressive brain disease and beyond."

CHAPTER 4
FEAR, THE VINYL FRONTIER

"SO, your Honor, the evidence will now clearly show how when fear controls the way we think, as an individual or collectively as a society, the results can lead to poor decision making which, in turn, if history repeating itself over and over and over is any guide, will more likely than not result in dire unintended consequences.

"To begin, it is important to note fear was actually *kneaded* in a primordial area of the brain referred to as the fear center or amygdala, (Mnemonic: Amy G. Dala), the purpose of which served a necessary role in helping our Distant Nomadic Ancestors (DNA) react to existential threats mostly having to do with predators with long pointy teeth, sharp claws, or poisonous fangs.

"Somewhere along the way, however, this important and necessary type of instinctual fear seemed to go the way of the dinosaur and was replaced by something we will be referring to as a postmodern, fabricated fear, which, for some, will look an awful lot like plain, old fashioned, ulcer-causing worrying."

"COUNSEL, explain to the Court more about the difference between instinctual fear and fabricated fear?"

"WELL, your Honor, the biggest difference between the two, in my opinion, is that the instinctual kind can be measured in real time as a reaction to what is perceived to be a real threat that has a definite beginning and a definite end.

"Whereas, fabricated fear, often a byproduct of an overly active imagination, tends to take on a life of its own and, therefore, by its very nature, keeps us bound to a perpetual state of anxiety so long as this particular type of fear continues to be fed by questions usually beginning with words like 'But what if...'

"And, your Honor, I believe fabricated fear was the type of fear being written about when it was said, 'Our fears are traitors, and make us lose the good we oft might win by fearing to attempt,' (William Shakespeare, 1564-1616).

"For the record, it is also important to note evolution probably only intended the release of just enough of the chemical cortisol from the adrenal glands to last for as long as it was necessary to help get past a clear and present danger and did not intend for us to suffer the unintended consequences of having too much of the chemical pumped into our system for as long as we choose to be animated in a perpetual state of fabricated fear.

"In a much broader context, your Honor, it is fair to draw a reasonable inference that when the general population itself becomes overcome with the same fabricated fear, the society itself is at just as much risk of suffering the unintended consequences of being trapped by fear as a person, especially when irrational fear turns into irrational anger, which if hate has its way can easily turn into irrational violence.

"It is important to note when the great Franciscan priest Richard Rohr warns us that what we are unable to transcend, we transmit. I would like to think he would agree that we must become more judicious when deciding where in the brain we choose to process thoughts so that transcendence can be spirit driven.

"So, your Honor, whereas an individual citizen can be viewed as a microcosm of the way in which a society suffers from the progeny of excessive fear, likewise, there are probably just many examples of where a nation could be perceived as a macrocosm of the way in which a citizen inculcates fear into the way he or she thinks."

"SORRY TO INTERRUPT your case in chief, Counsel, but do you now have an example in mind?"

"WHY YES, of course, your Honor, and not only am I prepared to show how a culture is as vulnerable as an individual when it becomes unable to transcend its fear and anger, I would even go so far as to say that that particular culture, if held to the same psychological standard as a person, might very well be diagnosed with a mental disorder."

"COUNSEL, please continue by sharing a familiar example."

"WELL, your Honor, the most obvious one that comes to mind—and one to which we can all relate—is how fear metastasized into anger and how our collective anger resulted in the violent act of invading Iraq without having had a rational pretext for going to war.

"More specifically, by watching the twin towers being destroyed over and over, it caused fear to burrow a hole into our collective consciousness, and caused any hope we might have had of thinking rationally to be sucked into the vortex of well-orchestrated, mushroom cloud imagery."

"COUNSEL, how do you intend to make an offer of proof that, if it were even possible, the country suffered a mental disorder as a result?"

"I WOULD LIKE to offer into evidence certain sections of the *Diagnostic and Statistical Manual of Mental Disorders (DSM-5)*, Fifth Edition, 2013, American Psychiatric Association, at page 659, where it could be argued our nation suffered an Antisocial Personality Disorder 301.7 (60.2) hereinafter referred to as APD) by invading Iraq."

"COUNSEL, let me stop you there and say it might be helpful to point out, the *Diagnostic and Statistical Manual of Mental Disorders (DSM-5)* is the gold standard used by psychiatrists and psychologists to diagnose mental disorders and is universally accepted as a credible authority.

"With that said, Counsel, let me start by asking you how many criteria are there to help in establishing an Antisocial Personality Disorder (APD) 301.7 (60.2); secondly, how many must be indicated before a clinical diagnosis can be made; and thirdly, how many of those criteria are you alleging were met using your example?"

"SO, your Honor, to answer your first question, there are seven separate criteria; to answer your second question, a patient need only exhibit three of these criteria in order for an Antisocial Personality Disorder diagnosis to be made; thirdly, the evidence will show the culture, which hereinafter will be referred to as the John Doe Nation, met all seven criteria when it invaded Iraq in 2003."

"COUNSEL, without taking too much time, please go over each criteria, and the Court will expect some legal authority as well."

"YES, your Honor, the first criteria of the DSM-5 for the John Doe Nation to be diagnosed with an APD occurs when it is shown there was a 'failure to conform to social norms with respect to lawful behaviors, as indicated by repeatedly performing acts that are grounds for arrest.'

"I would argue this first criteria was met, when the John Doe Nation breached the *United Nations Charter, Article 51*, of which the United States was a signatory, each time it attacked civilian populations without meeting the charter's requirement of only acting in self-defense or reacting to an imminent threat, which, for the record, sounds a lot like how evolution intended for us to react to instinctual fear."

"CONTINUE, COUNSEL."

"THE SECOND CRITERIA of having an APD, is 'deceitfulness, as indicated by repeated lying, use of aliases, or conning others for personal profit or pleasure.'

"Your Honor, the second criteria was met when the John Doe Nation lied about Iraq having Weapons of Mass Destruction (WMD).

"The third criterion of an APD, your Honor, is 'impulsivity or failure to plan ahead.'

"Your Honor, the third criterion was also met when the John Doe Nation went to war without planning a good way out. They left behind millions of displaced civilians, including small children, who must have had a lot of transfer trauma.

"The fourth criterion for having been diagnosed with APD, your Honor, is 'irritability and aggressiveness, as indicated by repeated physical fights or assaults.'

"Your Honor, I think the fourth criterion was met when the John Doe Nation repeatedly bombed civilian areas without discrimination, even though we knew or should have known that this would kill too many civilians, which is against Article 85 of the Geneva Convention, which the United States signed.

"The fifth criterion of being diagnosed with an APD, your Honor, is 'reckless disregard for safety of self or others.'

"Your Honor, the fifth criterion was met when the John Doe Nation knew or should have known the obvious risk his government was putting our future generations in by giving our enemies the predictable neuronal mimic reaction of wanting to get revenge."

"COUNSEL, was any legal authority violated with regards to the fifth criteria?"

. . .

"YES, your Honor, the Hague Conventions, Article 23, which, in part, forbids killing or wounding 'individuals belonging to the hostile nation or army' or 'to employ arms, projectiles, or material calculated to cause unnecessary suffering.'"

"PLEASE CONTINUE with your sixth criteria, and for the record, Counsel is using as his authority to allege a clinical diagnosis on a national scale, the *Diagnostic and Statistical Manual of Mental Disorders* (DSM-5), Fifth Edition, 2013, American Psychiatric Association, at page 659, for an Antisocial Personality Disorder 301.7 (60.2)."

"THE SIXTH CRITERION TO be diagnosed with an APD, your Honor, is 'consistent irresponsibility, as indicated by repeated failure to sustain consistent work behavior or honor financial obligations.'

"Your Honor, the sixth criteria was met when John Doe Nation depleted the United States Treasury of trillions of past, present, and future dollars while not meeting the financial obligations and needs of its own population, including, but not limited to, the needs of public schools, libraries, bridges, roads, housing, food, health care, hospitals, clean air and water, prenatal vitamins, soup, and showers for homeless vets, to name a few." (Cost Citation, www.nationalpriorities.org/cost.)

"FINAL CRITERIA, COUNSEL?"

"THE SEVENTH CRITERION TO be diagnosed with an APD, your Honor, is 'having lack of remorse, as indicated by being indifferent to or rationalizing having hurt, mistreated, or stolen from another.'

"Your Honor, the lack of remorse criteria is met, and, thus, the John Doe Nation runs the APD criteria table. It can be proven beyond a reasonable doubt that it has lost the ability to think about the human costs of having triggered the six previous criteria and the human costs of each, which, by the way, can be traced to a function of our orbital prefrontal cortex, which is where we learn our social values and probably keep our moral compass.

"So for the record, your Honor, this rather stark evidence was presented in order to dramatize how, if we allow fear to cloud our judgment, whether as a nation or as an individual who may be in the grips of Parkinson's panic, being able to make the correct choices regarding our health and safety in either situation may be illusory at best."

. . .

"FINAL THOUGHT, COUNSEL?"

"JUST THAT, your Honor, I would argue that if people get stuck in the fear and anger center of their brain, they should become aware they risk being able to only hunger and thirst for more fear and anger, but by the same token they should also know if they want to hunger and thirst for something more spirit driven, they must be willing to transition to another part of the brain by hungering and thirsting for something more humane." (Reference, Matthew 5:6)

"COUNSEL, sounds as if when people find themselves trapped in their fear center, for whatever reason, the only thing they have to fear is not enough fear."

CHAPTER 5

THE ONLY THING TO FEAR

"COUNSEL, I understand that before you leave the subject of fear, you want to impart a satirical historical event that showcases our collective fear in a more positive light."

"YES, your Honor, if the Court is willing to continue giving wide latitude to my poetic legal license, I could reference something having to do with recent discovered transcripts under an armoire in the Lincoln bedroom at the White House, which allegedly outline events leading up to Franklin Roosevelt's (FDR) first inaugural address in 1933, where he proclaimed, 'The only thing we have to fear, is fear itself.'"

. . .

"RELEVANCE, COUNSEL?"

"WELL, your Honor, these unverified transcripts will give the Court a more hopeful outlook regarding how we all have the power to use reason rather than fear when push comes to shove."

"ALL I CAN SAY, Counsel, is you are very fortunate all parties to this action stipulated to waiving strict compliance with the Federal Rules of Evidence; please proceed."

"WHAT THE AFOREMENTIONED discovery has revealed is that in leading up to the final draft of his 1933 inaugural address, where FDR said, 'The only thing we have to fear, is fear itself,' an earlier draft revealed the original address was a much wordier document where he was alleged to have said, 'The only thing we have to fear is fear of an out of control amygdala, resulting in way too much of the chemical cortisol being released from the adrenal glands, which can upset the balance of power between the mind-body complex.'

"With his newly appointed cabinet present, FDR was reported to have continued by saying, 'As dark clouds loom over the distant shores of Europe, we really must attempt, by all means necessary, to stop the flow of too much cortisol, the inflation rate of which stands the risk of leaving a synaptic chemical stagnation of toxic waste in its wake.

"'My fellow Americans,' the draft of the speech continued, 'I am as sympathetic to the way in which the sympathetic nervous system reacts to a stress hormone like cortisol as the next president, but we must all strive, at this time in our history to return to homeostasis, to a calmer place in our central nervous system.'

"The President elect, your Honor, a compassionate man, knew that this particular take on the 'fear' theme in the original draft was important, yet, as presented, was way too wordy and confusing. At the same time, he did not want to hurt the feelings of any members of his newly appointed cabinet, who may have had a part in penning this particular draft.

"According to the transcripts, FDR slowly moved away from the first draft and said, 'Okay people, love the speech; it's going to play well with many American families, especially as they gather around their hearths.

'Now I like paragraph one, line six, especially the part that says... We have nothing to fear! That really nails it; I like that part very much. It invites us to move back to our collective rational brain, where we, as a nation, are invited to problem solve and make the right decisions.

'The rest is good too, very informative, and says a lot about brain function, which will probably be understood and become more important in another generation or two, that is, if we don't stress ourselves out of existence. But, for now, since it's almost time for me to address the nation, I think we have to, don't take this the wrong way, it's just that, well, I think, for now, we have a more immediate need to be pithy, maybe a one liner about fear, maybe, let's start by thinking of something that rhymes, (rhyming plays well with democrats, they love catchy slogans).

'Okay, now we have about ten minutes left before we change the world. Let's put our heads together!

'Cordell Steward, you always have a thought or two?'

'Mr. President, the only thing I can think of that rhymes is, *The only thing we have to fear is beer*. That keeps the fear theme front and center and parses the sentence down to almost single digits and we have sort of a rhyme, more like a limerick, but the risk is it may not play as well in Boston or Chicago, this being so close to St. Patrick's Day and all.'

'Are you absolutely insane, Cordell?'

'Sorry for losing it, but we might as well join the temperance league, and lose the Irish vote to boot! Just what were you thinking?

'Hello people! When I say, think pithy, excuse my French diplomacy, but we have to be pithy without pithing anyone off!'

'Sorry, Mr. President, I'm better at foreign affairs.'

'That's okay, Cord, it's just that I'm just a little under the gun right now, with the world hanging in the balance, especially with all the alarming communiqués we have been getting from Eastern Europe and what have you.

'How about it, Frances Perkins, my Secretary of Labor, what you got, pretend you are back at Columbia University and show us how really smart people brainstorm.'

'Let me think, Mr. President; how, how about this: *The only thing we have to fear is fear in the rear of the hemisphere?* It kind of rhymes, fear, rear, hemisphere, if that's what you are really looking for, Mr. President, and it does incorporate a vague reference to the brain by using the word hemisphere.

'Good, good, Frances, just look at you. Who is thinking outside the oval box office? I'll tell you who. My new

Secretary of Labor, Frances Perkins, that's who is thinking outside the oval box office! Ha!

'How much time have we got left here? Three minutes!!! Okay, Fran, let's scrap the rhyme idea; take out the hemispheric brain reference; you're right, it's way too vague.

'We're still trying to pack in too much. It's got to be tight People!'

'Now you just relax, Mr. President. Knowing a bit or two about labor, since that is my department, I am making an executive order that you, Mr. President, take long, deep breaths.

'Okay, now that we have scaled down the phrase, taken out the rhyme, and kept the reason, the only thing we have to fear is, let me think, what comes after fear when it spirals out of control—a never ending faucet of fear.

'Let me think! It seems to me, Mr. President, the only thing we have to fear is being in a perpetual state of fear.'

'Wait a minute, Fran, how about something like, *We have nothing to fear, but never ending fear?*

'We're almost there. Think people! Fear is as old as the hills and not likely to go away on its own, especially if it remains faithful and true to its evolutionary purpose of being a reaction to an existential threat, instead of what scares me most, somehow allowing fear to last so long it becomes some sort of new-fangled misguided adaptive behavior.'

'Mr. President, if your greatest fear about fear is fear adapting into adaptive behavior, then you might want to tell the American people, 'The only thing we have to fear is fear itself.'

'By George Washington Carver, I think she's got it!'"

CHAPTER 6
THE PERILS OF PREJUDICE

You can sway a thousand men by appealing to their prejudice quicker than you can convince one man with logic.
—Robert A. Heinlein

"YOUR HONOR, a prejudice against some particular group or some particular activity, like daily exercise, more likely than not has its genesis within our stubborn insistence on thinking there is still a deep rooted primitive need to adopt and to protect a tribal mentality.

"It is, therefore, important not to underestimate the tenacious nature of prejudice, which burrows into the reptilian brain like a tick, whose primary motivation is to survive in the deep recesses of the human mind.

"There, then, may very well be a tribe of people with Parkinson's disease who harbor a pre-existing prejudice against a healthy diet and daily exercise, even to their detriment, indeed, still referring to those who render credence to such lifelines as 'health nuts'.

"Prejudice, in other words, can be explained as thought, processed in a more primordial part of the brain, that prevents us from connecting with our deepest identity, especially when we convince ourselves of the false narrative that someone or something, for some ambiguous reason, poses a threat."

"COUNSEL, please explain how people with Parkinson's might know if they have a prejudice against diet and exercise?"

"WELL, your Honor, the litmus test I would propose is whether a person somehow cannot get over the hurdle of judging healthy eating and stimulating daily exercise as being necessary evils, which, by the way, if they adopt that way of thinking, can expect little chance of having the staying power necessary to pursue the activities that would otherwise keep their brain cells alive."

. . .

"ANY SUGGESTIONS as to how someone can get over this particular hurdle, Counsel."

"WELL, your Honor, a person must perceive, and then truly believe, that diet and exercise are, instead, necessary blessings which have the power to keep brain cells alive."

"MOVING ALONG, Counsel, do you have an example of a person being able to overcome his prejudice?"

"DOES it have to be related to Parkinson's disease, your Honor?"

"YOU CAN USE ANY ILLUSTRATION, within reason, to prove that a prejudice is capable of being overcome to the benefit of the individual."

"WITH THAT IN MIND, your Honor, I do remember quite clearly being a percipient witness when a person fully overcame his racial prejudice.

"I might add, the experience I witnessed ties in well with the theme I have been pitching throughout these proceedings, which is, the best way to be healed from the toxic effect of a particular prejudice, or fear, is to gravitate and activate the rational part of the brain, where it can clearly be understood that 'Sunlight is the best disinfectant.' (Reference, Judge Louis Brandeis 1856-1941)

"It is from that part of the brain that it may also be understood that being held hostage to a racial prejudice results from suffering from a form of Post Traumatic Tribal Disorder (PTTD), which can be defined as lacking the capacity to disassociate oneself from the genetic slavery of ancestral racism.

"And when we are really honest with ourselves, we will someday come to realize that when a particular prejudice passes from one generation to the next, at some point in the family lineage, the prejudice is not as much held by the individual as the individual is held by the prejudice."

"COUNSEL, you mentioned that you had an example."

"YES, sorry, your Honor, Elwin Wilson was a young man in the early 1960s when he proudly wore the badge of being a self-professed bigot whose predatory prejudice of choice was having an aversion to those who were of a different color.

"Nearly fifty years later, Elwin Wilson had a change of heart, which was evidenced by the respect he showed for Congressman John Lewis, a civil rights legend, when they met on a stage at a Catholic university in California in 2009.

"This time, rather than spewing all manner of hatred and committing violence against John Lewis, as he had done in a bus depot in South Carolina in 1961, Elwin Wilson, humbled himself by asking to be forgiven for the sins he had once committed in his youth.

"Rather than following the modern trend of holding a person in his sin, Congressman Lewis decided to take the high road by releasing Mr. Wilson from the bondage of his transgressions by giving him a warm embrace and sending him on his way. (Dominican University, International Forgiveness Day, August 1, 2009)

"Your Honor, just as a neurological bookkeeping matter, I would just point out that the competing part of the brain to which Elwin Wilson would probably have had to gravitate and activate in order for him to have reaped the benefits of this particular healing experience was the orbitofrontal cortex which is found smack dab in a highly coveted part of the frontal lobe.

"Parenthetically, that is the part of the brain where neuroscientists believe social values are inculcated and where I personally believe our moral compass lies, waiting to be engaged.

"It is also worth noting Elwin Wilson passed not long after having made his peace with John Lewis."

CHAPTER 7
CRACKING COCAINE

"YOUR HONOR, probably the most competitive parts of the brain of all the competing areas of the brain is the one that is responsible for all of our addictions, which is the *nucleus accumbens septi,* a limbic system nucleus, which receives its input from yet another part of the brain referred to as the *ventral tegmental area* (VTA).

"As it was important to show how fear and prejudice could sabotage our ability to think rationally in order to make healthy decisions, the evidence will now show how an unhealthy addiction not only disrupts our ability to produce clear and reliable thinking, but it creates a physical dependency as well.

"And for our purposes, cluttering an already compromised brain with an addiction can become especially dangerous for those of us who suffer from a neurological disorder as invasive as Parkinson's disease, where, again, the primary use of our mental energy should be spent figuring out a way of keeping at-risk brain cells alive."

"COUNSEL, I will let you continue to develop your theme, but, for sake of judicial economy, I will allow you to use only one addiction to illustrate your point."

"THANK YOU, your Honor, citing only one addiction will actually be all that is necessary, since, as mentioned, all addictions, jointly and severally, initiate their activity in the same area of the brain found in that part of the limbic system."

"FOR THE RECORD, Counsel, again, what are the systems responsible for addictions?"

"THE TWO PARTS of the brain previously mentioned, your Honor, are the nucleus accumbens septi and the ventral tegmental area (VTA), which, I might add, are part of a system most neuroscientists refer to as the endogenous reward system and only seem to get out of control when there are not reasonable checks and balances initiated by the prefrontal cortex, to which there is a neural-pathway connection."

"WHICH ADDICTION WOULD you like to use, that is, Counsel, to illustrate your point?"

"I'D LIKE to take a crack at cocaine, your Honor."

"YOUR PUN, 'CRACK AT COCAINE,' reminds me of something I have been meaning to bring up, and speaking of addictions, it seems like an appropriate time to bring up your own addiction, where you can't seem to refrain from telling bad jokes."

"YES, YOUR HONOR."

"I WOULD FIRST LIKE to commend you on having shown great restraint, thus far, by not allowing tasteless humor to denigrate the sanctity of this Court."

. . .

"WELL, thank you, your Honor, I have been doing my best to keep my own personal addiction under control."

"COUNSEL, but I must add, when I heard you make the 'taking a crack at cocaine' wisecrack, I realized you may be at a tipping point.

"In light of this finding, as a pre-emptive measure, it might be a good time for me to rule that should you find yourself unable to control your own addiction to telling bad jokes, I am inclined to rule that you will be given just one opportunity to get all the jokes out of your own endogenous reward system at one time, and one time only, after which I would find it necessary to issue a gag order."

"THANK YOU, your Honor, forewarned is forearmed."

"GETTING BACK to the subject at hand, Counsel, where you were saying, addictions generally, and cocaine specifically, may work to sabotage the ability to make healthy decisions affecting our wellbeing, because, as you argue, they take thinking away from the rational part of the brain and direct it to yet another competing area of the brain."

. . .

"TO REVIEW, your Honor, the competing part of the brain that provides safe harbor for our addictions can be found in the endogenous reward system in the limbic system.

"More specifically, the endogenous reward system includes the VTA, which, coincidentally, projects the neurotransmitter dopamine to a specific part of the brain thought to control our desire for pleasure called the nucleus accumbens septi.

"Your Honor, it also should be mentioned that there is now corroborating scientific evidence there are neural pathways not only going from the VTA to the nucleus accumbens septi (where addictions are thought to take root), but also neuropaths projecting directly from the VTA to our prefrontal cortex (rational thought) and our orbital-frontal cortex (social conscience, sense of right and wrong, moral compass)."

"RELEVANCE, COUNSEL?"

"IT GIVES GREATER credence to an argument I would like to pitch, your Honor, that there becomes a greater probability of getting addicted to something unhealthy when the prefrontal cortex (rational thought) and/or the orbitofrontal cortex (moral compass) somehow get removed from the endogenous reward system's need for checks and balances.

"In other words, if all decisions having to do with what gives us pleasure are made exclusively by the nucleus accumbens septi, without the advice and consent of the prefrontal cortex and/or the orbitofrontal cortex, then, I believe it is only logical to assume the probability of suffering an unhealthy addiction becomes a clear and present danger.

"That's why, your Honor, if cocaine use is, indeed, under the exclusive control of the nucleus accumbens septi, without any frontal lobe checking and balancing, it's not likely the addict, on his own initiative, will ever say to an undercover cop, 'Whoa, dealer-dude, maybe it's time I reconsider whether it is in my best interest to use cocaine to trigger a feeling of intense elation by preventing dopamine from re-uptaking back into my ventral tegmental area just so I can stimulate my nucleus accumbens septi over and over, dude, cause I may be risking long term damage to the chemical integrity of my neurons and, besides, killing off brain cells could have the unintended consequences of blunting my emotional affect.'"

. . .

"MAKE your final point on this subject, Counsel, and let's move on."

"MY FINAL POINT, your Honor, would be that however a person chooses to deal with a progressive neurological brain disease like Parkinson's disease is a very personal matter.

"But I will say that if one expects to make sound decisions as to how to cope with a progressive brain disease, it stands to reason that good decisions are best made when the mind-body complex is not bogged down with any unnecessary addictions, including but not limited to, drugs or alcohol, and, instead, our mind and body are in strict compliance with the laws of mother nature.

"Because although she may be thought to be a nurturing parent, Mother Nature will turn on a dime if she catches anyone testing the limits of her naturally patented cellular brain signaling system which has been evolving for millions of years."

CHAPTER 8

A CELL WITH A VIEW

"YOUR HONOR, returning to our efforts to gain a better understanding of brain cells and the importance of keeping them alive, I would like to solicit the assistance of those who comprise the Court of Public Opinion, who may be willing to participate in an innovative experiment."

"WHAT DID you have in mind, Counsel?"

"IT IS ACTUALLY QUITE SIMPLE, and since participation will be done entirely on a voluntary basis, a person's right to privacy will not become an issue."

· · ·

"I NEED MORE DETAILS, COUNSEL."

"ALL I AM ASKING, your Honor, is that each member of the Court of Public Opinion contribute just one of their 100,000,000,000 (one hundred billion) brain cells, after which, each brain cell volunteered will be asked to vote and select the most popular neuron of all time to help us come to a better understanding of how a healthy human brain cell is supposed to function."

"HOW WILL the court be able to see something as small as a neuron?"

"THE BRAIN CELL SELECTED, if my experiment works, will be enlarged a million times by magnetic resonance imaging magnification."

"COUNSEL, since this whole idea may be the most ridiculous thing I've ever heard, is the Court correct in assuming, at this time, you want to exercise your one time option of ridding yourself forever of all your latent levity?"

· · ·

"YES, your Honor, and I apologize in advance if the humor falls below what is socially acceptable."

"DO WHAT IT TAKES, Counsel, but let the record reflect you are on notice you are exercising your one and only Parkinson's perk in the hopes you will exorcize yourself of this irritating and aggravating bad habit, which not only affects you but all the decent men and women within earshot of your questionable humor."

"THANK YOU, your Honor, I will do my best to make this experiment as educational and, I hope, funny as possible, but I trust you will be the judge of that."

"OKAY, Counsel, assuming you want me to play along, do I understand that if we are going to have some sort of cellular election, we need to continue these proceedings to a later date?"

"THAT'S THE THING, your Honor, in the world of a neuron, a brain cell gets more done in, let's say, a millisecond (.001 second) than a person gets done in a whole day.

"Just saying, from the time you consented to the experiment to the time you asked that last question, a cell with a view has been voted in almost unanimously by the neurons that chose to participate and is now ready to appear, assuming a certain condition is met."

"WHAT CONDITION IS THAT, COUNSEL?"

"YOUR HONOR, the brain cell elected will appear in court so long as a graphic illustrator captures it, and I quote the cell itself, 'One of my many good sides.'"

"COUNSEL, for now, let your celebrated witness, or, er, wit-cell, step up, er, move up to the witness, er, wit-cell stand, where the court clerk can swear him in."

"THANK YOU, but before doing that, your Honor, I would ask for your indulgence in granting me a short recess so a court-appointed artist can draw a medical legal illustration capturing the essence of the subject cell to assist the Court in its understanding of how a neuron works."

· · ·

"SURE, Counsel, it is about that time we took our morning recess anyway."

"BEFORE WE BREAK, your Honor, I have it on good authority that the brain cell of choice wants to know if it can sleep in a padded cell tonight with a bottle of *cell-tzer* on ice."

"ALL RIGHT, Counsel, I have promised to play along with your antics, but only to a point.

"With that said, I would be derelict in performing my duties on the bench if I did not admonish your so-called brain cell of choice!"

"YOUR HONOR, it agrees to behave, but adds that you would not be the first derelict to be admonished while occupying a bench."

"I CAN SEE where this is going, Counsel. Do you have an alternate wit-cell on stand-by you can call, that is, if this experiment gets out of hand?"

· · ·

"WELL, we do, your Honor, but I must tell the Court, the first alternate wit-cell suffered an injury after taking a punch to his cell body while starring in his last film."

"FOR THE RECORD, what is the name of your first alternate, Counsel?"

"THAT WOULD BE *CELL-VESTER CELL-LONE*."

"I SEE. "Are there any other alternates, Counsel?"

"JUST A COUPLE, your Honor, but I don't think they'd be any better."

"AND WHY WOULD THAT BE?"

"WELL, the second alternate is *Mar-cell Marcell*, but he refuses to say anything, and then, finally, there is *An-cell Adams*, who still insists on only seeing the world in black and white."

. . .

"OKAY, Counsel, but you are still on notice. The Court will have very little patience with a single, solitary, salacious cell that thinks it's a celebrity.

"Indeed, even as I speak, the bailiff has intercepted a note your wit-cell intended for certain members of the court staff, of the female persuasion, I might add, saying he, or it, wants to meet with them on the playground during our morning recess for purposes of being swung on a mood swing.

"For the record, Counsel, this is condescending and an affront to the Court as well, and I will not stand for it!"

"YOUR HONOR, my wit-cell agrees and, again, promises to behave, but seems to be concerned whether the *con descending* fell out of a plane."

"SORRY FOR INTERRUPTING COUNSEL, but let me read an important document the bailiff just handed me, marked 'Urgent!'

"For the record, it is a physician's report, whereby a court appointed forensic expert is of the opinion your wit-cell is competent to testify, but also warns the Court he will probably make the pitch that he should be excused because he suffers from the unproven psycholog-

JERRY HURTUBISE, J.D.

ical disorder, silly cell syndrome, once popularized amongst members of the Celtic community, who, over one hundred years ago, were credited with coining the phrase, 'What you are able to laugh at can't kill you,' and it might be helpful for some with Parkinson's to adopt this particular philosophy."

"YES, your Honor, being mostly of Irish descent myself, I am familiar with the fable of silly cell syndrome, which, by the way, no self-respecting psychologist would ever diagnose, no matter how much he or she believes laughter is the best medicine."

"COUNSEL, what are the symptoms of silly cell syndrome?"

"IT IS ALLEGED to be a rare mental condition, your Honor, occurring when an individual brain cell is somehow able to amuse other neurons with tasteless humor, one by one, until a disproportionate number of brain cells can't stop becoming amused at the world no matter how bad things seem to become.

"Some believe silly cells are the perfect antidote to plagues, pestilence, famine, war, and things of that nature.

"Getting back to the matter at hand, even now as his status of being a wit-cell hangs in the balance, he, it, attempts to amuse other neurons by continuing to perseverate on the *swing* theme, saying if allowed to spend extra time on the playground during the morning recess, he'll bribe a few *swing* voters to vote for you in your upcoming election, because from the looks of things, your Honor, your chances of winning on your own record do not look very appealing no matter how high the court gets.

"By continuing to perseverate on your Honor's upcoming election, he wants me to advise you to make better use of your spin cycle when whitewashing your dirty laundry, which, by the looks of it, police dogs are already starting to get wind of by sniffing around the courthouse.

"And now he wants me to warn you that if these curious canines start sniffing around your bench, he suggests you might want to start changing your briefs, and if that doesn't work, then you will be left with no other choice but to call in a swat team, who will not only give you the spanking you rightly deserve, but will also air your briefs in public. Better yet, to cut back on global warming, they will send your briefs directly to the stalls of justice where most of your opinions end up anyway."

"OKAY! Stop there, Counsel! I get it. Silly cell syndrome is somehow about getting a laugh by any means necessary in order to stave off anxiety and depression."

"PRECISELY, your Honor, but the good news is that cells that suffer from silly cell syndrome are for the most part harmless.

"It is just important to remember that although their humor may be funny at first, it doesn't take long before it just becomes irritating and aggravating."

"WELL, Counsel, as in your case, I am willing to give your witness a certain amount of latitude, but it or he, will, at some point, be expected to testify on some hard science to assist the Court in coming to a better understanding of how the human brain functions so people with Parkinson's will be able to make better decisions regarding their disease.

"Okay, then, with that said, Ladies and Gentlemen, it is now time for our morning recess."

CHAPTER 9

FAINT PRAISE

"WE ARE BACK on the record. Counsel, are you ready to proceed?"

"YES, your Honor, but, before I do, I would first ask the court clerk to mark this graphic illustration of my wit-cell as Exhibit One, after which time I will represent it is an accurate schematic drawing of the duly elected celebrity brain cell, Grouch-Cell Marx."

"LET it be marked and admitted into evidence as Exhibit One."

EXHIBIT ONE

Artist Rendition of Grouch-Cell Marx

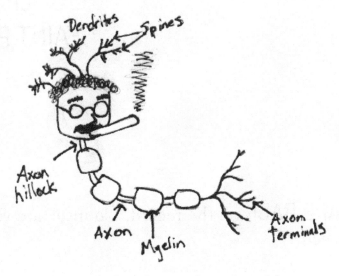

"I shot an elephant in my pajamas last night
and how he got there I'll never know."

For the Neuro-Scientist

"I shot a Lewy Body in my axon terminal last night
and how he got there I'll never know."

"Counsel, before you begin your direct examination of Grouch-Cell Marx, it might be helpful for you, again, to remind the Court how a healthy brain cell is designed to work."

. . .

"YOUR HONOR, to that end, I would submit to you the following outline:

'1. The space between brain cells, over which chemically charged 'information' passes, is called the 'synapse', thus comes terms like 'pre-synaptic terminal' and 'post-synaptic receptors'.

'2. Said chemical 'information' is transmitted across this synapse and when the neurotransmitters interact with receptors on the post-synaptic membrane, the chemical is converted back into an electrical signal, which propagates throughout the neuron that is next in line.

'3. Some neurotransmitters are 'excitatory', some 'inhibitory' and some, one in particular of great interest to us, 'dopamine' is both 'excitatory' and 'inhibitory', suggesting to me a respective transmitting 'key' only has the capacity to unlock a particular post-synaptic receptor to which it was evolutionarily designed to be compatible.

'4. I suspect that the type of 'dopamine' relevant in these proceedings, both 'excitatory' and 'inhibitory', loses more of the latter type of the neurotransmitter when neurons die, which would explain why tremors, inability to control movement, occur as frequently as they do.

'5. Again, with our earlier 'latch key kid' analogy in mind, the chemicals in the key (neurotransmitter) goes over the synapse and if the key fits, unlocks the postsynaptic receptor on the 'dendrites' which, are often described as what appear as tree branches or television antennas.

'6. The purpose of unlocking of the next cell 'lock' is, then, to open a portal through which a cavalcade of ions (charged atoms) flow freely into the user friendly cell, past the cell body, and to a place called the 'axon hillock' where it is determined whether the information is worthy of an action potential.

'7. Assuming the 'information' is worthy of an 'action potential', 'information' continues down a 'long' corridor, again, space is relative, called an 'axon', and although every synoptically charged event is measured in milliseconds, the more the axon is myelinated by support cells called oligodendrocytes ('myelin' is the material surrounding and insulating the axon), the faster the 'information' moves.

'8. It might also be relevant to mention that for any of this stuff to happen there must be a neuronal metabolism recipe of glucose breaking down and combining with oxygen in the mitochondria (Cell's Kitchen) to create the necessary energy."

· · ·

"THANK YOU, Counsel, you may begin with your witness."

"YOUR HONOR, I call to stand via magnetic resonance imaging magnification, Mr. Grouch-Cell Marx.

"Let me say, Mr. Marx, we are most honored to have you grace the Court by making your first appearance ever in these hallowed halls of justice."

"IT IS about time you fished me out of a jury pool where I must say I was swimming with much better looking sharks than what I see floating around in here.

"Imagine that, swimming with sharks who will probably get caught in a stingray set up by the State Bar for being so cell-fish with their attorney fees.

"I knew something was fishy when the sturgeon general came along and told us to get out of the pool for our own health and safety."

"OKAY, Mr. Marx, let's talk about your background."

. . .

"LET ME ASSURE YOU COUNSEL, I am not now, nor have I ever been, a member of the cognitive party and thus I refuse to testify until I'm promised a fifth, now that I think of it, any bottle the judge is hiding under his bench will do."

"COUNSEL, could you please assure Mr. Marx this is not the House Un-American Activities Committee, so taking the fifth will not be necessary."

"DO you understand what His Honor is saying, Mr. Marx?"

"SORRY, I was confusing witch hunts, but I will still insist the judge share whatever bottle he is hiding under his bench.

"Mr. Lawyer Sir, would you repeat the question and this time speak more slowly?"

"OKAY MR. MARX, just to establish you are competent to be a witness, do you have any degrees from any major universities?"

. . .

"STOP, Counsel, I will admit it! I'll come clean, if you just spare me the torment of your brutal cross-examination! It was me! I stole the oxygen that could have kept little Celia alive!"

"CELIA, MR. MARX?"

"CELIA THE SUFFOCATING CELL, I stole her oxygen supply after she had gone to all the trouble of breaking down glucose into lactate just so she could combine it with oxygen to cause a spark, but no, I took it all for myself, all I tell you, because there just wasn't enough for both of us, if only aerobic exercise was used to force more blood and oxygen into the brain, then there would have been enough for both of us, but no, oh woe is me!"

"MR. MARX, again, as the judge has promised you, you have not been summoned to this tribunal to be tried for any crime.

"The Court is well aware that since each one of us has billions of brain cells, no one is not going to quibble about losing a few neurons here and there, even if we refuse doing a daily regimen of aerobic exercise with the intent to restore normal signaling in the brain, which, arguably, might have saved the likes of little Celia."

"THAT'S the most ridiculous thing I have ever heard and, quite frankly, an affront to all Neanderthal neurons north of Nebraska.

"I would ask the judge to sign an order stopping you from making such a spectacle out of yourself and speaking of spectacles, where are my glasses so I can take a gander at Exhibit One.

"And after taking a gander, I might take two ganders and since they are free, maybe three ganders, it doesn't matter how many ganders I take because before long, we will have a flock of geese flying in here looking for a bench to make a mess of and then where will the judge be able to sit, but then again maybe he can take the stand like the rest of us?"

"GETTING BACK to my initial question, Mr. Marx, do you have any university degrees?"

"WHY INDEED I DO, funny you should ask just the way we rehearsed it, I have been given an honorary doctoral degree from Hebrew University of Jerusalem."

. . .

"WHY WOULD SUCH a prestigious university bestow upon you, ordinary brain cell, an honorary doctoral degree?"

"FOR THE DISCOVERY I made in the night sky."

"MY, my, what did you discover in the night sky Dr. Marx?"

"IT WAS THE TORAH BOREALIS."

"DID you win any award for making such an incredible discovery?"

"AS A MATTER OF FACT, I did, but it was nothing to write home about."

"WHY WAS THAT?"

. . .

"THE AWARD WAS ONLY A CONSTELLATION PRIZE."

"NONETHELESS, Dr. Marx, there must have been a banquet in your honor."

"WELL, Counsel, if you must know, there was, and it was held at a swanky hotel in the horse-racing capital of America."

"LOUISVILLE, KENTUCKY?"

"NO, FILLY-DELPHIA."

"THE CHEF MUST HAVE PREPARED a gourmet dinner, Dr. Marx?"

"I'LL SAY, he served filet mignon, which, by the way, I couldn't reach."

. . .

"WHY COULDN'T you reach the filet mignon, Dr. Marx?"

"THE STEAKS WERE TOO HIGH."

"NOT BEING able to eat your dinner must have made you feel dizzy."

"NOT NEARLY AS DIZZY as all the faint praise I was being given!"

"SURELY THERE WERE many famous people at such an event."

"I DO KNOW that Joe Montana was sent an invitation."

"DID HE ATTEND?"

"NO, HE DECIDED TO PASS."

. . .

"WHO ELSE WAS INVITED?"

"JERRY RICE."

"DID Jerry Rice come to your banquet?"

"NO, but he said he could make the reception."

"OKAY, Counsel, Dr. Marx, I think the Court has heard more than its fair share of humor for now."

"YES, your Honor, the Court has been more than generous with its time."

"DOES that also meet with your approval, Dr. Marx?"

"YES, Judge, especially since I was running out of material faster than handicapped parking at a Parkinson's convention."

. . .

"OKAY, Counsel, Dr. Marx, let's move on to something else after we take a short break so you can collect your thoughts."

"I WOULD RATHER COLLECT some money so I can buy a one way ticket back to my endogenous reward center where I belong."

CHAPTER 10

EXERCISING IS AN ACT OF LOVE

"DR. MARX, before I allow Counsel to continue with his direct examination, I would like to know what you discussed with Mr. Cultura during the break."

"WELL, first of all, he was curious about what happens biochemically within his brain when he triggers an aerobic high while exercising on his elliptical machine."

"WHAT DID YOU TELL HIM?"

"I TOLD him he sets off a virtual biochemical electrical firestorm the likes of which the Fourth of July has never known."

. . .

"DO you think aerobic exercises cause programs in the brain to work more efficiently, Dr. Marx?"

"YES."

"CAN YOU CITE AN EXAMPLE, Dr. Marx, where you think a person can intentionally set in motion electrically induced activity in a specific area of the brain, let's say in the basal ganglia?"

"I COULD CITE a million of 'em, Judge."

"JUST ONE WILL DO, DR. MARX."

"WELL, when a person engages in any premeditated aerobic activity with the intent of inducing a runner's high, it has the effect of setting in motion, within a brain cell, the loading of tiny vesicles containing the chemical dopamine, which is found in the presynaptic terminal.

"The purpose of which is so the neurotransmitter, dopamine, can be discharged into the synapse (space between neurons), after which time the vesicle circles back in order to reload more biochemical movement information and will continue doing so as long as it senses a particular movement is necessary."

"VESICLE, DR. MARX?"

"YEAH, Judge, vesicles can be thought of as little cargo ships that carry the dopamine that releases movement information from one cell to another cell, knowing full well this routine will be repeated over and over so long as there is an incentive for a person to keep moving, in the case of the basal ganglia, his arms and legs.

"And, personally, I am of the opinion this process of loading, discharging, and reloading chemical information will go on for as long as the movement is being waged because the vesicle is somehow programmed to think it is playing a vital role, first and foremost, in some important survival issue."

"AND IF THESE vesicles become unseaworthy, Dr. Marx, can this be problematic?"

. . .

"YES, things do get dangerous when other cargo ships go the way of the Titanic and block the corridors of these *vesicles*. In this case, they become debris and get in the way of vesicles that are still able to repeat the process of unloading and reloading important chemical information."

"DR. MARX, just to see if I got this right, the shipping process of little cargo containers, which you refer to as vesicles, is designed to assist in the navigation, more specifically, in our case, of motion information by somehow opening up and projecting it, said data, into the space between the brain cells, and they, vesicles, stand ready, if necessary, to reload more biochemical information and repeat the process for as long as movement is deemed important and they remain seaworthy."

"AND, I might add by way of an example, when Counsel premeditatedly attempts to induce an aerobic high on his elliptical machine, he is forcing the 'if necessary' part of your equation into a reality, *de facto*, setting in motion an 'all hands on deck' moment in the life of a vesicle and, thus, the argument could be made that a seaworthy *vesicle* will continue to sail so long as it has reason to instinctively believe it has a purpose driven life cycle.

"In my cellular opinion, if this is an accurate description of what amounts to a biological coming and going rule, a person with a neurological disorder, such as Parkinson's disease, may greatly benefit by initiating and, thus, setting in motion a certain chemical action in order to help insure this particular operating system continues to function.

"Otherwise, it would seem to make sense, the resilience of vesicles being able to load and reload important chemical information may have less of a chance of survival if they remain dormant.

"Sensing no motion is necessary just might be one of the reasons why, on a molecular level, these vesicles sense the role they play in the life of a cell is no longer of any value, break down from lack of use, and simply end up gumming up the system." (References, *Wild-type monomeric a-synuclein can impair vesicle endocytosis and synaptic fidelity via tubulin polymerization at the calyx of Held,* Kohaku Eguchi et. al, Journal of Neuroscience, June 2017; and *Autoimmunity May Have Role in Parkinson's Disease,* Catherine Paddock PhD, Medical News Today, June 21, 2017)."

· · ·

"ANYTHING YOU WANT to add to your example, Dr. Marx?"

"NO, Judge, other than to emphasize, again, that I suspect the vesicle example is but one thread in the tapestry of neuronal reactions set in motion in the brain when a person chooses, electrochemically, to play a more proactive role in the destiny of his or her brain cells by unleashing the power of a serious daily routine of aerobic exercise." (Reference, John J. Ratey, M.D., *Spark, The Revolutionary New Science of Exercise and the Brain,* New York: Little Brown and Company, 2008.)

"DR. MARX, getting back to the conversation you had with Mr. Cultura during the break, what else did you talk about?"

"WELL, in addition to trying to induce an aerobic high every day, he did have quite a bit to say about foods, some of which he believes are healthy for the brain and others of which he feels tend to sabotage our efforts to keep brain cells alive.

"Believing, then, that there is good glucose and bad glucose, which somehow finds its way into brain cells through the foods we eat, ultimately help either to keep neurons alive or leave the ill equipped to stay alive in order to fulfill their evolutionary destiny."

"DR. MARX, did he tell you specifically which foods pass the smell test and which do not?"

"NOT IN ANY DETAIL, but I could tell he wasn't a big fan of sugar, most saturated fats, or processed foods and was a huge fan of green leafy vegetables, eggs, sweet potatoes, avocadoes, broccoli, walnuts, beets, blueberries, strawberries, and foods rich in omega-3 like wild ocean salmon.

"All he would say beyond that was that if a person has enough interest in their diet helping to protect brain cells, all he or she has to do is get on the internet and type in 'good foods for the brain' and, probably more importantly, type in 'bad foods for the brain' and their dietary habits, hopefully, will never be the same.

"He also added, however, that since most people are very territorial when it comes to what they eat, the quickest way to put up a wall is by telling a person what he or she can and can't eat, especially by saying they should not eat so many foods giving them immediate gratification, a fact, by the way, which probably has not been lost on corporate executives in the food industry when marketing their products."

"DID that cover all the conversation you had with Mr. Cultura regarding diet, Dr. Marx?"

"HE DID SAY, for some, how critical it is to consume only digestible friendly foods so as to assure a successful morning constitution, particularly warning those who eat too much meat may have some interesting unintended consequences."

"I DON'T THINK we'll go there; what else did Counsel talk to you about during the break, Dr. Marx?"

"IN ADDITION to diet and exercise, he talked about some of the supplements he has experimented with taking."

. . .

"DID he say why he experimented with various dietary supplements?"

"WELL, he said that he believes that when a brain cell dies, it is, depending on the person whose brain cells are dying, probably the result of either a single proximate cause or many proximate causes.

"Nonetheless, since he does not believe science has enough information yet to know what exactly is causing brain cells to die in each different person, each potential proximate cause needs to be treated as a prime crime suspect until it is ruled out.

"So, to hedge his bet, he says he treats each of the billions of brain cells he still has as separate units and tries to make a list of all the different ways something can possibly go wrong and then determine whether there is a specific supplement that deals specifically with that particular proximate cause."

"PLEASE, Dr. Marx, read into the record the names of all relevant dietary supplements to which Counsel referred during the break."

. . .

"OBJECTION, your Honor, I must make a plea to the Court that Dr. Marx is not allowed to disclose the list of my dietary supplements, with which I have experimented at various times."

"WHAT IS the basis of your objection, Counsel?"

"YOUR HONOR, other than such a disclosure would violate my right to privacy, Parkinson's disease is obviously multifaceted and very personal to each person who has been given its diagnosis, and, quite frankly, my concern would be not knowing what the chemical reaction would be if the dietary supplements were to be taken in conjunction with prescribed medications already being taken by a person.

"Prescription drugs and supplements might, in other words, work at cross purposes and have a detrimental effect, especially on the person who has, up until now, taken drugs exclusively as his or her way of treating the disease."

"AND WHAT, Counsel, might those cross purposes be?"

· · ·

"WELL, your Honor, the way I see it, the purpose of taking supplements is to address specific problems so they might restore or protect the structural integrity of a brain cell so it might continue to live a healthy life in order to fulfill its evolutionary destiny of signaling vital information, in this case, motion.

"And medications being taken to curb symptoms of Parkinson's, as I understand it, do not purport to restore or protect the structural integrity of brain cells but instead pass through the blood brain barrier in order to replicate what these brain cells would otherwise have done but for their untimely death."

"COUNSEL, I see your point, but my ruling is to allow Dr. Marx to state for the record any and all supplements you mentioned during the break, but I will, to allay any of your concerns, also suggest, in no uncertain terms, that since these supplements may be at odds with a medication regimen being taken by a person being treated for Parkinson's, the order of this Court is that such a person taking said prescribed medications get permission from his or her medical doctor before taking any supplements hereinafter mentioned.

"Now, Dr. Marx, please state for the record the supplements Counsel mentioned to you during the break."

. . .

"PREDICTABLY, Judge, there was the usual list of suspects; magnesium, zinc, vitamins B, C, D, and E, usually found in a multivitamin, but Counsel also included other supplements intended to target specific brain issues: Alpha Lipoic Acid (which purports to have antioxidant activity, helping to fight free radicals), phosphatidylserine (which purports to support a healthy membrane surrounding the brain cell), CoQ-10 (which purports to support cellular energy production), NAC, i.e., n-acetylcysteine (which purports to help the brain produce glutathione, a super important antioxidant for the brain's protection from oxidative stress caused by too many free radicals) and Vinpocetine (which purports to support cognitive performance by increasing blood circulation)."

"WAS he more specific regarding why he experimented with, let's say, phosphatidylserine?"

"WELL, he did say he believes that this particular supplement bolsters and supports the membrane surrounding each brain cell, and if the reason a person is losing brain cells is because he or she is particularly vulnerable to suffering the consequences of messed up membranes, then this specific supplement may be something useful."

. . .

"DID he explain more about why he thought it might be useful?"

"YES, because a healthy membrane has a lot to do with how ions, charged atoms, interact with one another inside and outside a brain cell, and this, he thinks, is important because controlling just the right amount of ionic balance between ions from within and without a neuron determines whether the brain cell remains in a resting state when appropriate or when it's time for temperatures to rise and for there to be an action potential.

"And without a healthy membrane safely regulating the highly evolved ionic charge differential between ions inside and outside the neuron, he has bought into the theory that such an anomaly can cause an abnormal electrical discharge resulting in things like tremors or slowness of motion (bradykinesia)."

"WAS that a complete list of supplements Counsel told you about?"

"JUST THE ONES I CAN REMEMBER."

· · ·

"WAS ANYTHING ELSE DISCUSSED, DR. MARX?"

"HE DID MENTION, he spends most of his day staying one step ahead of his Parkinson's by using his elliptical machine, which he refers to as the great equalizer, as well as taking long walks and doing online fitness classes."

"WHAT DID he mean by the great equalizer?"

"I ASKED HIM THAT, and he said, 'When I get going on my elliptical machine, with my eyes closed, after a spell, the movement of the machine takes me to a place where for one magical moment every day I am free of any disability."

"DID you discuss anything else with Counsel, Dr. Marx?"

· · ·

"WELL, he did begin to explain how much more beneficial and healthier it is to breathe through your nose and deeply into what feels like your tummy, like a baby naturally does."

"DID he actually use the word tummy, Dr. Marx?"

"I SWEAR he used the word tummy."

"WHY DID he say it was important to breathe through your nose and into your tummy?"

"WELL, Judge, he didn't but, instead, changed the subject."

"WHAT DID HE SAY, DR. MARX?"

"FOR SOME REASON, he thought it was important for all to hear that intense aerobic exercise intent on keeping brain cells alive can easily be perceived as an act of love."

. . .

"DID HE OFFER AN EXPLANATION, DR. MARX?"

"HE, in all earnestness, felt that if those with Parkinson's truly understood the pain and anguish, often hidden, suffered by those who love them and take care of them, they would exact any means under their control in order to stay as healthy as possible, for as long as possible, in order to soften the sorrow of those whose devotion they, probably, would freely admit they do not deserve, but nonetheless, by the grace of God, have been blessed."

"I SEE, Dr. Marx is again your witness, Counsel."

"THANK YOU, YOUR HONOR."

CHAPTER 11
BRAIN DICE

"DR. MARX, I would now like to change directions by having you explain to the Court how we can all better understand human brain functions by, maybe, likening the brain to something to which we all can relate."

"WELL, let's see, I suppose you could think of the human brain as an institution of higher learning."

"WHAT WOULD you like to call this institution of higher learning, Dr. Marx?"

"HOW ABOUT WE call it Brain-Dice University?"

. . .

"WHY BRAIN-DICE UNIVERSITY?"

"ASIDE FROM BEING a clever play on words, it will remind us that by luck of the conceptual draw, the strengths and vulnerabilities of each of our brain cells are in large part the result of a genetic lottery (nature) and the environment into which we have been planted (nurture)."

"PLEASE CONTINUE, Dr. Marx, and if you could, where possible, please help us to understand your explanation in the context of the testimony already received into evidence."

"WITH THAT IN MIND, Brain-Dice University, or BDU, like other highly rated universities, relies for its life or accreditation on a constellation of factors, including having highly evolved interconnected pathways to various departments, a well maintained infrastructure, and a thriving administration to oversee its operations.

"For illustrative purposes, each department at BDU can be likened to a different brain function.

"And in order for a university or human brain to maintain its accreditation with the outside world, various departments (different brain functions) have evolved to the point where subspecialties within each department have come to exist that are accountable to a highly evolved administration (frontal lobe).

"Trouble, however, can erupt when a specific subspecialty of a particular department thinks it can act autonomously outside the purview of other departments (parts of the brain) or administrative offices (the frontal lobe).

"As the evidence has shown, this can happen when the ventral tegmental area (reward system) attempts to assert its independent authority when an addiction convinces the department of which it is a part (limbic system) that it can go solo (resulting in loss of self control), especially when there is an absence of any oversight from that part of the administration (prefrontal cortex) overseeing such matters.

"Another example of this type of departmental mutiny, in evidence, is when the amygdala (the anger and fear center) insists, again, absent reason, on perseverating over and over and over... on a future fear, which almost never happens because perpetual panic is usually not based upon any credible truth."

. . .

"DR. MARX, could you give examples of how a particular department at BDU can be likened to a distinct brain function?"

"YES, certainly not an exhaustive list, but let's say a few of the different departments might be : Department of Visual Arts (occipital lobe), the Department of Memory, Emotion, and Learning (limbic system), the Department of Truth and Reconciliation (orbitofrontal cortex), and, what is most important to us, the Department of Motor Movement (extrapyramidal motor programs and the pyramidal motor system)."

"EXCUSE ME FOR INTERRUPTING, Dr. Marx, but it might be helpful for us to know what distinguishes extrapyramidal motor programs from the pyramidal motor system?"

"YES, of course, the pyramidal motor system plans, initiates, and executes (PIE) a movement directly to the spinal cord, whereas the extrapyramidal motor programs can be thought of as highly evolved departmental subspecialties, e.g., the basal ganglia, which does not connect directly to the spinal cord and, therefore, must pass movement information through the motor cortex.

"Which, by the way, results in us doing unconscious things like swinging our arms freely while walking (substantia nigra in the basal ganglia) or consciously learning a new skilled motor movement (cerebellum)."

"THANK YOU, DR. MARX; PLEASE CONTINUE."

"IT SHOULD ALSO BE EMPHASIZED that BDU can only exist if it has a highly evolved Maintenance Department (the brain's reticular formation), which keeps all the students or brain cells alive without them having to worry about important housekeeping matters, e.g., the heart beating, breathing, and blood flowing.

"And, predictably, the Administration Department at Brain-Dice, already mentioned, has evolved to the prime, most enlightened areas of the brain, the frontal lobe, best known for being able to calculate, calibrate, and inculcate evolutionarily friendly executive decisions, sound judgments, and organized planning."

"DR. MARX, although we have earlier touched upon the subject, can you now talk about how brain cells at BDU are able to pass along vital information within and beyond the particular department to which they have evolved?"

"ALTHOUGH, for the most part, brain cells work the same way, some have short axons, which are creatively designed to be able to transmit information interdepartmentally (inside a nucleus itself); whereas other brain cells have longer axons enabling them use connective or association pathways to project information inter-departmentally (between nucleus')."

"I'M SORRY, Dr. Marx. For purposes of review, can you define for the Court what you mean by the word axon?"

"AN AXON IS that long extension part of me; for identification purposes, take another gander at Exhibit One, which facilitates the transmission of electrically signaled information to my brother and sister cells, at least to those which have applications able to receive compatible information and, thus, are able to understand the information I am trying to communicate."

. . .

"THANK YOU, Dr. Marx, now you are saying some brain cells stay in their own department and others send their impulses outside their respective department."

"SO, some brain cells, students at BDU if you will, just want to project their information locally, that is, within their own department, and others want to pass along information more globally, keeping in mind that all information has to pass a strict scrutiny test monitored by department heads of each department, whose postgraduate degrees in evolution have earned them a chair in the highly coveted cerebral cortex."

"AGAIN, I'm sorry, Dr. Marx, but can you define cerebral cortex?"

"YEAH, it's the most recent part of the brain to have evolved, a thin outside layer of the cerebrum, which, at Brain-Dice can be thought to be the place where axons of each department hook up with their respective department heads, who, in turn, have the final say as to what information gets transmitted."

· · ·

"WITH YOUR DEPARTMENT head analogy in mind, can you cite some examples, Dr. Marx, of the specific places in the cerebral cortex where department heads understand the appropriate language of their respective departments?"

"WELL, yes, there are places like the cingulate cortex, that part of the cerebral cortex that is closely aligned with the limbic system and therefore programmed to speak the departmental language of Memory, Emotions, and Learning (or MEL-ish).

"The prefrontal cortex, although more administrative, is programmed to speak many dialects, including the language of solving problems and making executive decisions.

"The motor cortex, which, as we have learned, is programmed to speak the language of conscious and unconscious movement, and, again, when too many brain cells die in a certain part of the basal ganglia called the substantia nigra, it can end up causing Parkinson's.

"The primary cortex and a related department, the somatosensory cortex, are programmed to speak the languages of pain and touch.

"Yet another example would be the ventromedial prefrontal cortex, programmed to speak the language of being able, hopefully, to make sound judgments like seeing how treating a movement disorder with movement may make a lot of sense for someone who has Parkinson's disease."

"NOW DR. MARX, since we are interested in staying on point by hearing testimony as it relates to the disease of Parkinson's, can you expand upon how brain cells pass information to the department head who chairs the motor cortex at BDU?"

"WELL, again, I can't say it too many times, but I might remind the Court that the thing about Parkinson's is that its root cause can be traced to a very specific part of the midbrain located in the basal ganglia called the substantia nigra, where, by the time of an early diagnosis of the disease, more or less about half the brain cells in that particular part of the brain have died off.

"The good news is that at the time of being diagnosed, a person's substantia nigra brain cell glass is, again, still about half full, many of whose neurons are still capable of being saved, that is, assuming the person diagnosed is willing to take the lead on center stage and be willing to play more than a cameo role."

. . .

"DR. MARX, might that role have something to do with a disciplined approach to daily aerobic exercise and a proper diet?"

"EXCUSE ME FOR THE INTERRUPTION, Counsel, but I will not allow Dr. Marx to simply regurgitate what, no doubt, has probably been received into evidence multiple times already, which would make his testimony on this matter cumulative."

"COULD YOU BE MORE SPECIFIC, your Honor?"

"THE COURT, Counsel, already knows from prior testimony, this witness, more likely than not, will suggest restoring life to remaining brain cells in order to take a stab at keeping Parkinson's at bay. First, this is in large part contingent upon committing, routinely, to an aerobics regimen in order to induce an athletic high so as to restore normal neuronal signaling in all parts of the brain, including, but not limited to, the basal ganglia and its related parts, most specifically, the substantia nigra.

"Secondly, he would probably repeat the testimony that the consumption of doctor approved brain supplements might go a long way in helping to repair the pre-existing damage done to the structural integrity of brain cells, so long as it can be determined why a particular part of the brain cell is indeed vulnerable, when and if that becomes possible.

"And, thirdly, I don't want him to repeat that simply by going to the internet and finding 'best foods for the brain,' and, probably more importantly, typing in 'worst foods for the brain,' a person can in some way aid and abet the healthy life of a brain cell.

"So unless Dr. Marx has anything left to add to that particular line of questioning, let me assure you, Counsel, the Court gets it, so it suggests you move on to something else."

"YES, your Honor. Dr. Marx, moving along, assuming hypothetically that Judge Soloman was correct in his assessment as to how you were going to respond to my last question, is there anything you would like to add?"

"JUST THAT WE would be well advised to learn something physical therapists have known for a long time."

"AND THAT WOULD BE, DR. MARX?"

. . .

"BY ANALOGY, let's say a particular part of the knee has been damaged beyond repair.

"Sometimes, healthier, more user-friendly parts of the knee, surrounding the compromised part, are often able to be strengthened to the point where they are able to offer aid and comfort to the overall health of the knee, making it a whole lot easier to move."

"DR. MARX, I can understand how this would work with a knee, but can you give the Court an example of another part of the brain that could be developed that might help a person with Parkinson's disease?"

"AN EXAMPLE WOULD BE to engage the incredibly adaptively learned skilled motor behavior of another motor program in the brain called the cerebellum."

"DR. MARX, what is the function of the cerebellum and what is its relevant nexus with Parkinson's disease?"

. . .

"THE CEREBELLUM, home to about half of our brain cells, is found at the base of the brain and controls coordination of voluntary movement, gross and fine motor skills, posture, and balance.

"Indeed, it is a learned, skilled motor movement machine, cranking out more pathways than a well landscaped retirement community.

"And it is important for people with Parkinson's to know about the insatiable appetite the cerebellum has for refining movement, the importance of which is illustrated when a person gets on an elliptical machine for the very first time.

"Initial sensations on such a device will often result in feeling foreign as one experiences the new-fangled sensation of arms and legs moving simultaneously.

"Some may be so overcome by the fear of falling that they give up, which may result in the cerebellum never being given a chance to work its evolutionary magic of helping to define newly learned skilled motor movements.

"This would mean never discovering that still within their quiver are learned skilled motor survival skill arrows genetically bred to adapt, literally, to any new environment, simply by activating humongous candelabra-like dendrites referred to as Purkinje cells."

. . .

"COUNSEL, excuse me for interrupting, but perhaps this is as good a time as any to take our afternoon recess and when we get back, we can wrap up the testimony of Dr. Marx."

"COUNSEL, we are back on the record, and I would like to know how you want to finish up with this witness?"

"YOUR HONOR, I think it would be best to end the testimony of Dr. Marx on a lighter note by having him explain to the Court what happens on a biochemical level when we attempt to use humor as a way of lifting our spirits."

"SO BE IT, Counsel; I agree, it might help to end his testimony on a lighter note; please continue."

"FIRST, Dr. Marx, what happens chemically in the brain when someone hears a joke, assuming it is funny?"

. . .

"WELL, when a person hears a joke that makes him or her laugh, the endogenous reward system is stimulated, and dopamine is released, which causes pleasure.

"That is why when someone is asked, sometimes, what he or she likes most about another person and the response is, 'They make me laugh,' what is actually being said by the person answering the question is that he or she enjoys the pleasure of being stimulated by the dopamine being released in the ventral tegmental area of the brain."

"YEAH, Dr. Marx, but what makes something funny?"

"MOST PEOPLE, because of how their brains are wired, enjoy hearing something that is out of the ordinary, something unexpected."

"PLEASE EXPLAIN."

"WELL, we might be going along, minding our own business, having certain expectations that the events in our lives unfold in a certain order, and that is exactly the way things are supposed to happen from the perspective of the parietal and temporal lobes of the brain.

"And then some wisecracker comes along and says something out of the ordinary that disrupts our normal view of the world and how it is supposed to be perceived, and for some reason, when it is done creatively in a harmless way, it can make us laugh by moving us to the reward area of the brain, and that seems to be a positive experience so long as the joke stays within the bounds of what is socially acceptable."

"DR. MARX, can you experiment on us by attempting to move us from the parts of the brain where we normally perceive reality to the reward area by telling us, let's say, the first twenty jokes that come to mind?"

"SURE, let's see. Let me start by saying that there is nothing particularly funny about seeing Monet in a swimming pool, but what moves that particular perception out of the ordinary and, thus, might be funny, is when it is learned that in the pool, one of the greatest artists of all time, is doing the brushstroke.

"Likewise, there is nothing funny in and of itself for a ballet company to have a patron saint until you learn the patron saint is Bishop Desmond Tutu.

"And staying on the ballet theme, there is nothing unusual about the fact a ballet dancer gave a good interview until it was revealed she gave a good interview because she stayed on point.

"Sticking with the arts, a person going to the jazz festival is not funny in and of itself until you learn the person going to the jazz festival got there by taking the 'coal-train'.

"Getting back to the swim theme, there is absolutely nothing funny about a swim team going to a swim meet until a person finds out the way they got there was by carpooling.

"And a person might actually be surprised to learn that I would take my financial advice from my gardener until he or she learned the gardener knew a lot about hedge funds.

"It was the same gardener who couldn't step out of his garden because he had planted his feet.

"A person might also find it funny to learn that when the scientist combined milk and oxygen, he was the first to discover dairy air.

"By the same token, some might think their reward system has hit the jackpot, upon learning the reason the Dalai Lama went to Las Vegas was because he wanted 'to bet'.

"But, by the same token, there will probably be only modest stimulation of their reward system upon learning poker players do not make great hikers because they like to shuffle.

"Changing lanes, although a car can't feel it, but the way it would feel if it could feel after going cross country without a muffle would be exhausting.

"Which reminds me that the reason most car mechanics seldom get sick is because they are auto immune.

"And that most runners never get depressed because they take things in stride.

"And let's not forget the best meal to have on Ash Wednesday is lentil soup.

"And the reason why the saint could not understand why God gave her a halo was because it was over her head.

"Speaking of food, two jokes ago, it should have been obvious that a body builder's favorite type of seafood is mussels.

"And speaking of speaking, when the fog came back to San Francisco, it said, 'I mist you'.

"Also, let's not forget that what Rip Van Winkle insisted upon before he got married was a pre-nap.

"Or when toddlers want to have a good time, they have a 'poddy,' and what is probably funnier is that a person from Boston may not understand why toddlers wanting to have a 'poddy' is funny.

"But that same person from Boston might laugh when you tell him or her that the last thing the queen does before she leaves the bathroom is a royal flush.

"That's twenty, Counsel; would you like twenty more?"

"NO, for some reason I no longer wish to be an accomplice to the telling or hearing of questionable humor.

"But I would like to thank you for your testimony, Dr. Marx, and that is all I have for this witness, your Honor."

"YOU MAY BE EXCUSED, Dr. Marx, but before you leave, is there any advice you would like to share with those who suffer from a progressive brain disease?"

"YES, JUDGE."

· · ·

"WHAT ADVICE WOULD THAT BE?"

"IT IS important for them to know that if things get rough, they should always be like the morning dawn."

"HOW CAN a person who suffers from a progressive brain disease be like the morning dawn, Dr. Marx?"

"BY MAKING DEW, your Honor, by making dew."

"ON THAT NOTE, you are now excused, Dr. Marx."

CHAPTER 12

THE ONE-LEGGED STOOL

"COUNSEL, how do you wish to proceed?"

"YOUR HONOR, I would just like to proceed by saying using prescription medications as the exclusive means of treating Parkinson's disease makes about as much sense as trying to sit on a one-legged stool."

"PLEASE CONTINUE."

"AS THE COURT has already been made aware, there are other ways of helping to treat Parkinson's disease other than by just taking drugs and drugs alone.

"To review, if the objective is to restore as much structural integrity to a brain cell as possible so that it lives longer, in my humble opinion, that particular goal depends mostly upon the recognition of the powerful effect diet and exercise have on the life of a neuron.

"The traditional medical paradigm, at least until recently, has relied almost entirely on making and using a Frankenstein-like version of the neurotransmitter dopamine. This version is meant to bring back to life a certain part of the brain by doing what natural dopamine was supposed to do in the part of the brain we are most interested in (the substantia nigra).

"And to its credit, this amazing science has been able to do so quite effectively for many of its users, but still, at the end of the day, no known drug purports to help to keep brain cells alive in any way whatsoever or restore their structural integrity, so neurons can continue to function as they were meant to function.

"That is probably why drug dosage must escalate commensurate with the number of brain cells dying in that part of the basal ganglia we have learned is the substantia nigra."

"COUNSEL, please state for the record the names of different drugs that are manufactured as a way of replacing or replicating the neurotransmitter dopamine."

"YES, your Honor, since the list of synthetic brain drugs being marketed continues to expand to capture market share, it may, indeed, be better to focus the Court's attention on the two most popular medications that have been manufactured to date: (1) dopamine agonists, which claim to act like, mimic, or replicate dopamine, and (2) levodopa, which claims to synthetically be able to propagate itself into the actual dopamine by absorbing itself into the brain cell."

"COULD you expound more on the dopamine agonist, Counsel?"

"OF COURSE, first by saying, the purpose of a dopamine agonist is to act like or mimic what dopamine does by taking a shot and, presumably, inputting movement information with applicable postsynaptic receptors and dendrites, which are clearly visible on Exhibit One.

"This, I can only presume, is ambitious, since, of the trillions of postsynaptic receptors in the brain, successful dopaminergic (not a word I made up) input, under the best of evolutionary circumstances, is a challenge in and of itself that has taken millions of years to perfect.

"Again, no small feat for a bold young dopamine agonist, since, in addition to there being trillions of receptors, it somehow has to be able to know how to match excitatory sensitive keys (neurotransmitters) with excitatory sensitive locks (dendrites) and, if that wasn't challenging enough, somehow intuit that inhibitory sensitive keys (neurotransmitters), likewise, only fit into inhibitory sensitive locks (dendrites) in order to do things like prevent pesky tremors and keep us moving fluidly.

"But still, your Honor, in defense of this coming of age dopamine agonist, it would be patently unfair to hold this brave little toaster of a synthetic brain drug to the same gold standard set by evolution for the real dopamine.

"Which is probably one of the reasons why when the dopamine agonist doesn't hit the right receptors, it probably can cause more side effects than when there are Quakers at a peace rally."

"COUNSEL, speaking of side effects, are the side effects of levodopa and the dopamine agonist the same?"

· · ·

"THEY VARY A BIT, but they are mostly the same."

"CAN you read into the record some of the reported side effects levodopa has had for some people, Counsel, with the understanding most people who are prescribed these particular medications have few, if any, side effects?"

"YES, your Honor, if I may have a moment, yes, it is reported consumers are warned that when taking the most popular Parkinson's medicine, levodopa, side effects experienced, may include fever, stiff muscles, confusion, abnormal thinking, fast or irregular heartbeat, sweating, drowsiness, dizziness, lightheadedness, fainting, unusual gambling or sexual urges, constipation, diarrhea, dry mouth, headache, increased sweating, loss of appetite, nausea, taste changes, trouble sleeping, upset stomach, urinary tract infection, vomiting, suddenly falling asleep, blood in vomit, chest pain, hallucinations, involuntary movement, depression, anxiety, restlessness, irritability, sore throat, suicidal thoughts, spasms, blurred or double vision, rash, hives, itching, difficulty breathing, tightness in the chest, swelling of the mouth, face, lips..."

. . .

"COUNSEL, of all the side-effects just outlined, 'unusual gambling or sexual urges' seemed to jump out at me the most.

"Are you certain such ideations have been reported as side effects from taking this medication?"

"YES, YOUR HONOR."

"IS THERE any scientific explanation for how this happens, Counsel?"

"WELL, your Honor, the pharmacy only provides a list of potential side effects, not an explanation as to how the drugs might react chemically in the brain to cause such side effects."

"IN OTHER WORDS, Counsel, you don't have a clue as to how these excessive gambling or sexual urges are manifested in the brain in some consumers after having taken the drug."

. . .

"ONLY MY OWN un-peer reviewed theory, your Honor, which might, under different circumstances, be objected to as being speculative, to say nothing regarding my incompetence in rendering such an opinion."

"WITH THAT BEING SAID, since I suspect you are going to offer it anyway, let's hear your explanation, Counsel."

"WELL, your Honor, I am floating the hypothesis that when the drug is taken and finds its way into the brain of a consumer who is particularly vulnerable to triggering the side effect of either an excessive sexual or gambling urge, he or she probably, also suffers the side effect of not being able to reason because he or she for some reason becomes unable to access his or her prefrontal cortex for purposes of weighing and balancing.

"And if the Court buys this 'no frontal lobe' theory, it can be further hypothesized that when electrical and chemical neuronal activity becomes estranged from higher levels of cognition, another competing area of the brain will attempt to fill the void, here the endogenous reward system, which, presumably, if left unchecked, as we have learned from earlier discussions, can lead to all sorts of addictions."

. . .

"COUNSEL, getting back to the subject at hand, if the Court were to allow you to pose any question to the smartest pharmacologist in the world regarding the causes and effects occurring when a dopamine agonist stimulates physiologic activity at cell receptors normally stimulated by naturally occurring substances (dopamine), what would it be?"

"WOULD I be allowed to ask a compound question, your Honor?"

"SINCE STRICT COMPLIANCE with the Federal Rules of Evidence has already been waived in this hearing, Counsel, you have permission to compound your question to your little heart's content."

"WELL THEN, your Honor, I do have such a question that I would like to ask the smartest pharmacologist in the world. I am curious about whether our dopamine receptors in our postsynaptic membranes are transformed in any way when interacting with a synthetic brain drug like a dopamine agonist. Let's assume changes are made to the structural integrity of a brain cell, which I believe to be quite likely. I'd like to know how our own remaining dopamine reacts to the postsynaptic receptor after it has consummated a new marriage with a synthetic drug! And another thing, how would our own dopamine compete with a dopamine agonist for the same dopamine receptor in real time? If our own dopamine is unable to compete with a dopamine agonist, does the drug leave behind a calling card of toxic residue? If so, does the dopamine agonist clean up after itself? Or, perhaps it expects glial cells (the brain's janitorial service, numbering in the trillions) to dispose of the toxic residue into some sort of synthetic super fund site in the brain. And yet another question, if the relationship between the drug and the glial cells, somehow, becomes acrimonious, do glial cells (astrocytes) vote to go on strike leaving any alleged toxic residue free reign to create a breeding ground for free radicals to steal even more negative ions from unsuspecting molecules? Oh, and speaking of ions, does the dopamine agonist affect the way a cellular membrane regulates the delicate balance of how ions inside and outside neuron react with each other so as not to cause abnormal electrical discharges like hand tremors which are the crown jewel of all Parkinson's symptoms?"

. . .

"OKAY, okay, Counsel, sorry I asked, now tell the Court more about the other medication you mentioned, levodopa."

"SO, your Honor, levodopa was actually the first medication proven effective for treating a chronic de-generative neurologic disease, being absorbed into the bloodstream from the small intestines and traveling through the blood to the brain, where it is alleged to be converted into the active neurotransmitter dopamine." (Citation, *Parkinson's Disease: Medications*, 4th Edition, National Parkinson Foundation, 2011, p.8.)

"Levodopa, the big L-DOPA on campus, unlike the agonist, can't be accused of suffering from dopamine envy, since it claims to be able to convert itself into the real stuff by absorbing itself into the nerve cell.

"But unfortunately, like other contraindicated anti-evolutionary panaceas too good to be true, it was soon discovered levodopa would gradually, for most, lose its effectiveness at controlling symptoms of the disease when taken at the same dosage, coincidentally in tandem with how many brain cells were biting the dendrite dust, thus resulting in the inevitable consequences of a person having to take higher doses of the drug to compensate for the exponential neuronal attrition rate."

. . .

"COUNSEL, I understand you have prepared some sort of video to illustrate the point you are trying to make."

"YES, your Honor, I would now like to present an animation showing what it would be like if levodopa was pitted against Parkinson's disease in what I have dubbed 'The Fight of the Century'."

"WHAT IS ITS PROBATIVE VALUE, COUNSEL?"

"BY ENGAGING SENSES, the video intends to help the Court to come to a better understanding of the intended benefits and some of the shortcomings of the highly popular medication."

"YOU MAY PRESENT YOUR ANIMATION, Counsel, so long as the probative value outweighs any prejudicial effect. Someone please dim the lights."

"THANK YOU, your Honor, let the record reflect that I am now turning on the projector."

CHAPTER 13
HOPA L-DOPA

'HELLO SPORTS FANS, the stage has been set for us at the one hundred year old Rose Bowl in beautiful Pasadena, California, where the sun is setting over a restless crowd of people, new and old, most diagnosed with Parkinson's, whose lives hang in the balance as they prepare to watch how a tiny pill has agreed to go head to head with, dare we say, one of the fastest growing progressive brain diseases in the world.

'My name is Howard Co-cell and I am here, along with my sidekick, Bret Buddy-Berger, to bring you all the live action.'

'THAT'S RIGHT, Howard, the stakes could not be higher as the spotlight beams down to the center of the ring where hope in a little pill seems to burn eternally, that is, until there is a cure for the dreaded disease.

'It truly is the fight of the century. Our sound feed is hooked up. Let's go ringside and listen to the introductions.'

'LADIES AND GENTLEMEN, in the far corner, the odds on favorite to be in the medicine cabinet of most Parkinson's patients in America, weighing in at a strapping 100 milligrams, is the synaptic sultan of Sweden, the uncontested champion of all drugs fighting Parkinson's disease, the Levo-Legend, Leeeeeeeee-voooooo-dopa!

(Crowd heard screaming wildly as the pill disrobes and rolls in a circular motion around the ring.)

'And in the near corner, weighing in at 800 pounds, the grim weeper of those who do the hopa-dopa, the destroyer of mobility, the apprentice of apprehension, the Parkinson Pundertaker.'

(Crowd heard booing as brain disease stares beyond the crowd and into the sunset.)

'WOW, Howard, we've waited for what seems like forever for this brash little upstart of a pill to come along and make good on its promise of, I want to make sure I get the quote from the lightweight right, yes, here it is, 'To make pulp out of Parkinson's,' who it simply calls 'P' since it wants to, again, 'Abbreviate the hell out of the disease,' excuse my French toast.'

'SORRY TO INTERRUPT, Bret, but it looks like the champ and the Pundertaker seem to be jawing at the center of the ring even before the fight begins.

'One thing for sure, I would not like to be the one getting between the pugilistic pill and the dreaded disease at this particular moment!'

'I KNOW, Howard, can we turn the volume back up, from here it looks like this vociferous little drug is now rolling around P in a circular fashion, trash talking, not feeling the least bit intimidated by a disease that promises to leave hundreds of millions in its wake before they find a cure, and speaking of wakes, wake me when this one is over.'

'NOW, now, there's no need to bail on me now, Bret ole buddy, last I looked, we weren't taking on water, at least not yet.

'Can we get some feedback at ringside, let's listen in and hear what the heck is going on as it looks like the pugilistic pill is eyeball to eyeball with the only 800-pound gorilla in this room, what's that, we're hooked up now, let's listen in.'

'YOU ARE THINKING of taking me down, P; there isn't any other dopa-meaner in the ring, so you must be thinking of taking me down.

'That's right, P, you're the only clown going down because, say it, 'The champ is a mover, not a shaker; a mover not a shaker; a mover not a shaker....'

'OH HOWARD, the crowd loves this spry little guy, who is, reportedly, the odds on favorite medication to be willing to stand up, forgive me for repeating, to what some health care professionals are calling the most tragic and fastest growing progressive brain disease in the history of world, promising to turn lives inside out and outside in.'

'WELL, Bret, there the Champ goes, now taunting P, as if he was a hummingbird, as the old disease, or should I say relatively new disease, is now lumbering back to its corner for a few last instructions from a trainer who needs no introduction, Dr. Dementia or as he is better known in pharmacological circles as Double D.'

'THAT'S RIGHT, Howard, if you can believe the beat writers, it's no secret Double D has been grooming this relatively new disease since at least the industrial revolution suggesting there is some pretty convincing evidence there is an environmental connection between industrial pollution, especially pesticides, and Parkinson's disease, at least for some.'

'POINT TAKEN, Bret, but let's not forget, some of our corporate sponsors still dispute the 'pollution factor' and would prefer we stick with 'genetic predisposition' as the primary talking point as to who is at most risk for getting Parkinson's.'

'I AGREE, Howard, rewind, rewind, well anyway, circling back, even though training sessions are closed to the public, I heard, Double D did give the beat writers some fat to chew on.'

. . .

'YEAH, I know, Bret, Double D said it's not so much about P being able to punch the lights out of the Champ, but more about the Pundertaker just waiting around and letting brain cells self-destruct on their own even as the pill is used, 'All in good time my pretty, all in good time.'

'And since the pill doesn't do a thing to keep brain cells alive, P has all the time in the world to just let the Champ dance around the ring weaving and bobbing, stabbing and poking at P, using up juice, until one day the once feisty pill becomes a thing of the past and the patient has to take more drastic measures like upping his medication or going the way of a deep brain stimulation surgery. (DBS)'

'A REAL SHAME, Howard, that no one has figured out how to stop the disease in its tracks.'

'THAT'S RIGHT, Mr. Buddy-Berger, Double D did let it slip; P will easily be able to hang in there with the champ for as long as it takes, just by taking pill punches to its dendrite receptors, which, for all the hoopla, at the end of the bout, doesn't change the fact brain cells just keep dying off.

'Supposedly, you didn't hear it me, Bret, but the skinny is P is using the champ as a chump, a distraction, by letting the pesky pill control the narrative so long as it distracts people from thinking about what really has the best chance of keeping brain cells alive in the substantia nigra, which of course is diet and exercise.'

'WHOA, Howard, let's back up, 'substantia-Nigeria what?' Who, here, is biting off his 'nasal ganglia' to spite his facial masking.

'One of us in the booth might as well tell them to hold the mayo at the Clinic, so move over C. Everett Kooping Cough and make room for a guy who sounds like he knows what the hell-o is going on in the four lobes of the human brain.'

'I KNOW, Bret, look at me, mom, I'm not really a doctor, but I'm playing one on television!

'Seriously, Bret, let me just finish my thought by saying that word in the neuro-burrow is that P knows that each levodopa pill lasts three, maybe four hours per pill, max, so the fix is on to have other pugilistic pills just keep lining up to be taken; it doesn't matter a bit to P.

'All P knows is that all this extracurricular activity is taking the attention away from figuring out a way of keeping the home fires burning in the brain cells that are left to fend for themselves, and that's exactly what's happening when a person doesn't take diet and exercise seriously to help keep the fire stoked.

'In other words, there is an oven in each brain cell (mitochondria). Most call it a furnace; I like to call it an oven because, in better times, it is where a brain cell could easily whip up an energy soufflé.

'But Double D also let it slip, P can easily handle pill poppers in any match day or night, any place, any time, as long as that is all they do, but is scared to death of cellular oven light pilot starters, people priming the pump with aerobic energy and eating foods that are glucose friendly.'

'WOW, Howard, I agree; it sounds like this diet and exercise thing you keep harping on can work for some people; otherwise, it might as well be game, set, and match for P even before the opening bell rings.

'That is so long as a person doesn't let fear, a prejudice or an addiction cause him to act like a deer in headlights.'

. . .

'YEAH, Bret, too bad, but it sounds like the only magic bullet fans of the champ are willing to take is the one to the cell body.'

'BUT STILL, Howard, I should mention that, even as we speak we're getting quite a bit of fire on the wire from our sponsors, who still believe, the feisty little fireplug of a pill offers hope for the hopeless, that is, until there's a cure, which they keep promising is right around the corner.

'Don't you agree with our sponsors Howard, that the pill offers hope to the hopeless, that is until they find a cure, preferably one maximizing not only health but shareholder profits as well, a true win-win situation?

'Don't you agree, it's best to hope for a win-win, Howard, are you still with us, Howard, Howard, you still with me, do we need to take a break so our local stations can identify themselves?'

'I'M SORRY, Bret, it just struck me that if the purpose of hope is to spring eternal, its commitment, then, can only, at best, reflect faintly against a darkening night sky, casting just a tint of purple hue against the San Gabriel Mountains surrounding us, left only, almost betrayed, Bret, by what soft light still lingers from a waning pastel

145

covering the horizon, which by simply promising a new dawn, it knows not to be true, seems to be a cruel fiction.

'But, Bret, even now, as the stars are being hung, my heart sings from a softer, more translucent hymnal, almost a longing, a kinder resolve for those who suffer only in the fire of hope, a knowing they need not know darkness only in enmity of a night sky, but of a new gestation, a flowering of the morning glory promising to give the day a new, truly, more vibrant fragrance leading to a more lasting and deeper sense of health and, yes, a fuller sense of mortality.'

'WHOA, hey come on, Howard, take a few deep ones, big guy, let's get down off that moonbeam, the fans want smash mouth sports talk, we are here for a fight, not a Polly Anna bonnet sonnet.'

'SORRY BRET, I just don't know what came over me.'

'WELL, sports fans, let's take a commercial break, so my pal Howard can get grounded.

'We'll be right back after a word from our sponsors, who know that bringing good things to life means being able to appreciate a good joke from time to time, like Howard

146

here trying to put one over on us by going all Henry David Thorough-fare.

'Three, two, one, we're off the air.

'Howard, my friend, I do hope we have a 'toast' clause in our contract, because I got a feeling that is exactly what we are.'

CHAPTER 14
DEATH OF A CELL, MAN

"COUNSEL, before you continue, I have a question with regards to something you just implied in your animation.

"It was suggested there is an oven or a furnace in each brain cell—the mitochondria, I think you called it— where a brain cell creates a chemical reaction somehow giving it the energy to do what it is intends to do.

"And when a threshold number of brain cells in a part of the basal ganglia are no longer capable of creating this chemical reaction, they risk certain death, and that puts a person at greater risk of getting Parkinson's disease.

"It sounds to me, Counsel, you are suggesting Parkinson's is the result of a brain cell having a faulty furnace, whereas throughout these proceedings you have made every effort to implicate other reasons for causing the death of brain cells, which, in turn, you argue may cause the disease."

"YOUR HONOR, IS THERE A QUESTION PENDING?"

"WELL, yes, Counsel, before I get to it, based upon the Court's own research and a summary of the various reasons for which you have raised on your own, I have chronicled some of the ways a brain cell can die.

"And it would seem, each way, standing separately, can be implicated in causing the death of cells in numbers substantial enough to cause or contribute to a diagnosis of Parkinson's disease.

"Counsel, the list of ten you are already floating includes:

1. A damaged brain cell membrane making it challenging to safely regulate the highly evolved ionic charge differential between ions inside and outside the neuron;

2. Abnormal accumulations of clumps of a protein called Lewy bodies gumming up the inner workings of a brain cell;

3. A major link between gut microbes and Parkinson's; (Citation, Michael S. Okun, M.D., *Gut Bacteria and H.pylori,* Parkinson Report, National Parkinson Foundation, Spring, 2017.)

4. Your own theory which suggests a brain cell can die from biochemical oxygen deficiency (BOD);

5. The malfunctioning of microscopic cargo ships (vesicles) charged with loading and unloading the payload of the neurotransmitter dopamine (information) in the space between cells and then circling back to reload new information;

6. The related subsequent stockpiling of discarded vesicles, again, gumming or what you would call gunking up the system, turning an information highway into a vehicular nightmare; (References, *Wild-type monomeric a-synucleusn can impair vesicle endocytosis and synaptic fidelity via tubulin polymerization at the calyx of Held,* Kohgaku Eguchi, et. al, Journal of Neuroscience, June 2017; and *Autoimmunity May Have Role in Parkinson's Disease,* Catherine Paddock PhD, Medical News Today, June 21, 2017.)

7. When astrocytes, neuronal 'nannies' outside the neuron, are no longer able to clean up the toxic mess a brain cell leaves behind; (References, *Neurotoxic Reactive Astrocytes Are Induced By Activated Microglia,* Nature, International Weekly Journal of Science, 481-487, Jan.

26, 2017, in *Aberrant Astrocytes May Lead to Parkinson's*, J. Fernandes, PhD, parkinsonsnewstoday.com, Jan. 20, 2017.)

8. Free radicals, alleged to be cannibalistic molecules, stalking the brain terrain like zombies in hopes of regaining a lost negative ion, usually at the expense of other, more healthy molecules, which has the effect of turning them into zombies as well;

9. Brain cell ingesting bad glucose, e.g., high glycemic foods, rather than good glucose, e.g., low glycemic foods, making neuronal metabolism less efficient;

10. Finally, let's not forget another theory you are also peddling, that the ongoing pumping of the stress related chemical cortisol resulting from being in a constant state of manufactured fear reduces our immunological capabilities, which may also result in the death of brain cells.

"And now, Counsel, you are pitching what sounds like yet another theory of causation, where you claim to be linking a faulty furnace in the brain cell (mitochondria) to Parkinson's disease, without even as much as a citation linking a faulty mitochondria to Parkinson's.

"So my question, Counsel, is, which of all your so-called theories is the one you are implicating as the one causing the disease?"

. . .

"NO DISRESPECT INTENDED, your Honor, but your question assumes facts not in evidence by inferring there is only one cause for why a threshold number of brain cells die, which leads to a diagnosis of Parkinson's disease.

"And, secondly, it is also an incomplete hypothetical in that it does not specify as to which person in the Parkinson's population is the subject of your inquiry since the reason for losing brain cells may differ from individual to individual since what causes the disease more likely than not varies depending upon the patient being examined.

"In other words, for one person, his or her brain cells might have remained healthy but for faulty mitochondria; for another, healthy brain cells may have been compromised by defective membranes; for yet another, healthy brain cells may have been compromised by a collapse in the cellular system outside the neuron, e.g., gut microbes or no longer functioning astrocytes; and so on and so forth. And where it really gets dicey is when a person's brain cells may have remained healthy, but for a combination of some or all of the causes you listed, to say nothing of those yet to be discovered.

"Not properly providing credible authority alleging a link between faulty mitochondria and Parkinson's disease was an oversight, and I do respectfully apologize to the Court. (Citations, *Mitochondrial Function and Autophagy: Integrating Proteotoxic, Redox, and Metabolic Stress in Parkinson's Disease*, Jianhua Zhang, PhD, Center for Free Radical Biology, Department of Pathology, University of Alabama at Birmingham, Department of Veterans Affairs, Birmingham VA Medical Center, January 17, 2018; and *Mitochondrial Biology and Parkinson's Disease*, Celine Perier and Miquel Vila, Cold Spring Harbor Perspectives in Medicine, February 2, 2012.)"

"NO DISRESPECT TAKEN, Counsel. Please continue with your focus on the legal theory of proximate cause and how it relates to Parkinson's disease."

"WELL, your Honor, looking at Parkinson's through the lens of a lawyer, as I just argued, I strongly suspect that the cause of why brain cells are dying in one person diagnosed with the disease may be entirely different for another person diagnosed with the same disease."

"DIFFERENT CAUSE OR CAUSES, same disease diagnosis?"

. . .

"EXACTLY; in other words, it is my position that a brain cell may die for known and, probably, many still unknown reasons depending on the particular neuronal vulnerabilities unique to the individual being diagnosed.

"Each diagnosis also has unique genetic, environmental, and dietary components to factor into the equation as well.

"Your Honor, there should be no mystery as to what causes Parkinson's since the disease is so closely linked to a great number of brain cells dying in a particular part of the brain in the basal ganglia, which we have marked as the substantia nigra.

"Again, the tricky part is figuring out why these brain cells are dying at such an alarming rate, and, thus, I humbly suggest the cure will depend upon how to keep brain cells alive or, in the alternative, whether science can somehow figure out a way of developing new neural pathways (neuroplasticity).

"Coming full circle to the issue of proximate causation, then, as it relates to Parkinson's disease, it is best understood in the context that the disease is triggered when a threshold number of neurons, for whatever reason, die in an area of the brain that does not allow molecular information having to do with movement to pass electrochemically between brain cells and out into the muscles.

"The challenge before this court is understanding that although the symptoms of Parkinson's manifest themselves, for the most part, similarly in people diagnosed, it cannot be overemphasized that what causes the death of brain cells, resulting in the disease, again, may vary from person to person depending upon the particular vulnerabilities of their respective brain cells."

"COUNSEL, am I correct in assuming the answer, then, to the question of what is the proximate cause of Parkinson's disease, would in large part depend upon who is being examined and the discovery as to why his or her respective brain cells are dying, and based upon those particular neuronal vulnerabilities, it might follow that at risk brain cells may lose their capacity to function for any number of reasons, including, but not limited to, a cell's faulty furnace (mitochondria)?"

"YES, your Honor, and until there is a cure, we must do everything in our power to play an active role in helping to keep them alive."

CHAPTER 15
THE LEMMING TREE

"SO, your Honor, the best way of keeping my own brain cells alive, includes, in part, incorporating into my daily routine an intense aerobic exercise therapy, where I attempt to stimulate a chemical reaction in the brain so as to restore normal signaling.

"And by doing this every day, I have found it not only has the added benefit of giving me a sense of wellbeing, often causing a feeling of ecstasy, but also has the lucky strike of assuring me a healthy sleep at night, so long as I don't nap during the day.

"Deep sleep, then, along with diet and exercise, all working in concert, I believe, all have something very important to do with the ongoing maintenance of healthy neurons as well as restoring the structural integrity of at-risk brain cells on the brink of destruction."

. . .

"SO WHAT YOU ARE SAYING, Counsel, is that intense daily aerobic exercise might help those who have a problem sleeping at night?"

"NO PUN INTENDED, but that would be a blanket statement, but again, your Honor, it would depend on the individual and what is preventing him or her from getting a good night's sleep.

"For example, some with Parkinson's might find their sleep troubles have something to do with the fatigue they suffer, which results from taking a medication that causes them to become drowsy, and they think they need to nap during the day.

"If, let's say, your Honor, a drug prescribed for Parkinson's has the side effect of causing a person to be sleepy during the day to the point where all he or she wants to do is nap, then, obviously, that person's motivation to exercise will also be affected until it becomes a vicious cycle of napping during the day and counting sheep at night.

"Instead of napping, a person may want to fight the temptation by becoming physically active in some way until, like a cloud in the sky, the fatigue passes, which, I guarantee, it always does

"And, speaking of the importance of sleep at night, I might add that it is in deeper REM level slumber that a person can venture into some rather epic dreams, which has the added benefit of being able to clean out the psychological cellar of excess baggage hidden deep within the subconscious."

"COUNSEL, tell us more about one of your so-called epic dreams."

"WELL, your Honor, I don't want to bore the Court, but I will say I do have a recurring dream where I come to a better understanding of how the brain can be used for either good or evil since that is what I seem to perse-verate on during much of my waking hours."

"TELL the Court about this recurring dream you have, Counsel."

"IN GENERAL, it is about a shadowy character by the name of Otto Cratt whose purpose in the life of my dream, it would seem, is to create enough fear in people so they think only he can protect them from harm when, in fact, the only protecting they need is from him trying to control their mind and resulting behavior.

"In other words, this figment of my shadow side is hell bent on convincing his followers of a big lie, which just happens to be in vogue at a particular moment in history, even though it could never pass a strict scrutiny test if tested in a court of law since it is always low on evidence and high on hype, but, nonetheless, each time it is told it adds more fertilizer to his lemming tree."

"IF HIS UNTRUTHS are short on evidence, Counsel, why are the people in your dream inclined to put their trust in him?"

"WELL, I am not sure, but I do know he promises his followers, the lemmings growing on his lemming tree, he can stop any pain the truth might be causing by keeping them away from the rational part of their brain, and, instead, they are encouraged to process thought from a more reptilian part where they simply become low hanging fruit on his poisonous tree.

"Otto Cratt, in other words, has an uncanny knack of being able to convince his legions of lemmings to join him in an unholy alliance by promising them power, prestige, or possessions in exchange for simply allowing him to move the truth as far away from their moral compass firmly implanted in the orbital frontal cortex.

"In my dream, when the alliance is consummated, Otto Cratt takes control over the life of another by putting truth on a conveyor belt to be reprogrammed, until the truth becomes whatever he wants it to be."

"COUNSEL, does this recurring dream always follow the same script?"

"USUALLY, your Honor, but there is, however, one version that does stand out, where a character named Bratman goes on a mission to stop Otto Cratt from being able to grind the truth in the machinations of our mind."

"IF YOU CAN BE BRIEF, it might be relevant for you to share that particular version of your dream with the court, Counsel."

"YOUR HONOR, I would think any probative value of my sharing of my dream would be greatly outweighed by the embarrassment I would suffer before fellow members of the bar by disclosing that particular version, which, by all accounts, is just a lot of dream debris."

"COUNSEL, the probative value of evidence is usually weighed against the prejudicial effect it might have, not by how much embarrassment it causes a lawyer who obviously has already tested the limits of social and legal etiquette in these proceedings.

"So my order is that you describe, as best you can, the version of your recurring dream where, I suspect, you are somehow trying to rid the world of the likes of this Otto Cratt fellow."

"WELL, it is against my better judgment, since the dream itself is so fragmented and often nonsensical, but if it is what you order, I would simply ask the Court for its permission to allow me to read into the record that particular version, which I have chronicled in a dream journal I have been keeping since being diagnosed with Parkinson's disease."

"THAT WILL BE FINE, Counsel; now proceed."

· · ·

"WELL, your Honor, this version always begins with Bratman coming upon his sidekick, Bratboy, who is in some apparent distress.

"Bratman starts by saying something like, 'Whoa, whoa, whoa, Bratboy, you look as though you just lost your best brat friend, what's doing?'

"That is when Bratboy responds, 'Well, Bratman, if you must know, I tossed and turned all night long after hearing Otto Cratt attack you on the radio by saying, 'Old school, more seasoned intellectual brats, like the great and powerful Bratman, still insist on using their frontal lobe no matter how much pain the truth reveals.'

"Then, Bratman, Otto Cratt goes on to say that since the fate of your big fat brat brain is already sealed, because of all the brain cells you lose every day, you might as well concede defeat and park your bratty butt on a couch in front of a big screen television, until your brain turns into, dare I repeat what he said, yes, I must, until your brain turns into, into, no, I can't, I just can't say it aloud...'

'SAY IT, Bratboy, did Otto Cratt use the fiendish "B" word? Did he fill the airwaves with the "B" word in order to create a nightmarish neurological association?

'What were his exact words, tell me, you little brat, tell me!'

'WHAT OTTO CRATT SAID, Bratman, is that, over time, with age, all brat brains, no matter how much they align themselves with the truth, will enter into a lower level neurological mish-mash-mush zone, and will turn into...'

'SAY IT, BRATBOY!'

'...IN the end, even your brain, Bratman, will turn into, 'Bratwurst'!'

'THERE, there, now, Bratboy, take a few deep big bad brat breaths and don't get caught up in Otto Cratt's web of perpetual primordial panic.'

'I KNOW, I know, Bratman, but what's a gullible little brat to do when the reptilian receptors of Otto Cratt wrap their tentacles around my more primitive fear based neurotic neurons?'

. . .

'I'LL TELL you what a spirit driven little brat like you is expected to do, he is expected to use his free-will by pushing his mental pedal to the metal and choosing, instead, to use that part of his brat brain designed to inculcate critical thinking skills.

'And by doing this, the truth will set you free by exposing how activated nascent neurotic neurons, trapped in the reptilian brain, are easy prey for him and those like him, who know full well that by continuing to keep us locked into a constant state of irrational emotion or fear, he can advance the fragmented figments of his fanatical fantasy for fame and fortune.

'Now damn it, you already know this Bratboy!'

'HOLY-TURNING-OVER-TABLES-IN-THE-TEMPLE-OF-THE-TEMPORAL-LOBE, Bratman!!! I seem to have jump-started a raw nerve in the well seasoned seat of wisdom in your orbitofrontal cortex.'

'I'M SORRY, Bratboy, especially for modeling parental indignation in a way that may later be mimicked by the brain cells in your cerebral cortex, where it is believed long term memories are stored.'

'But how many times must you and your bratty friends be reminded that even the humblest of brat brains come equipped with a frontal lobe capable of all the biochemical electrical dischargeable fire power necessary to zap the connections being made by the likes of Otto Cratt between neurotic neurons and reptilian receptors?'

'HOLY- HELL- CELL- IN- BRAT- BASKET, Bratman! What I hear you saying is that someday, just maybe, when courage overcomes cowardice, the progeny of Otto Cratt will no longer be able to lead children of the brat into any more damn brain-to-bratwurst brat traps.

'Sorry for using profanity for dramatic effect, Bratman, but brain cells in my frontal lobe are already beginning to get pretty damn, I'm sorry, pretty darn sparked up around the notion that brains of brats may someday be able to evolve to a point, especially if dietary and aerobic discoveries are made in time, where brat brains never stand the risk of turning into bratwurst!'

'HERE, here, my profane little gluten free brat cracker, even as we speak, the modern trend already suggests there is credible scientific evidence suggesting diet and aerobic exercise have a lot more to do with keeping brain cells alive than most brats could ever imagine.

(References, Amy Berger, MS, CNS, NTP, *The Alzheimer's Antidote,* White River Junction: Chelsea Green Publishing, 2017 and John J. Ratey, M.D., *Spark, The Revolutionary New Science of Exercise and the Brain,* New York: Little, Brown and Company, 2008.)'

'HOLY-CLOUDS-OF-DIETARY-AND-EXERCISE, justice moves slowly, if it moves at all, Bratman! Please tell me you're not suggesting that brats like me around the world are already able to improve their mind-body complex simply by consuming more in the way of good foods for the brain and less in the way of bad foods for the brain, while, at the same time, chasing the holy grail of aerobic exercise, the coveted runner's high, tell me it isn't so!'

'STEP aside you non-believing little brick-o-brat, so other more evolved little brats might make better use of their four lobes and two fissures in order to feed a world starving for more in the way of dietary and aerobic truth.'

'I'M sorry for a momentary primordial leap of faithless disbelief, Bratman, but you must tell me how I too can get started on the neuropath less traveled so I too can help feed a world starving for attitudinal change.'

'YOU MIGHT BEGIN, Bratboy, by remembering a mnemonic, which will, as prophesied by the ancient brat masters, remind brats of all ages of the relationship between diet, exercise, and the positive effect they can have on certain neurotransmitters that have to do with mood, learning and motivation.'

'PLEASE, Bratman, do tell, do tell me the mnemonic, a mnemonic probably so clever, it will forever remind children of the brat the names of those particular neurotransmitters, the depletion of which may cause anxiety and depression so severe a brain cell might be at risk of losing its beta-bing beta-boom.'

'WELL, well, well, three-holes-in-the-ground, Bratboy, I can see you are finally willing to take your dendrites to a place where they have not yet dared to be discharged, maybe even to a place where you may learn good diet and proper exercise should be looked upon with gratitude, which is an attitude that should have been a beatitude.

'So, then, the depleted neurotransmitters, which can be considered prime suspects in causing anxiety or depression when they become biochemically challenged, in some cases, due, in part, to such variables as bad diet and no exercise, are: <u>S</u>erotonin (mood, appetite and perception), <u>A</u>cetylcholine (learning and memory) and <u>D</u>opamine (motivation and anticipated pleasure) or 'SAD.'

'HOLY-BRAT-IN-THE-BRONX, Bratman, tell me how I too might become aerobically possessed, so I might free myself from these dastardly bio-chemical imbalances in the brain.'

'YES, I will indeed show you the neuropath of most resistance to neuronal inflammation and oxidative stress, my budding overachieving aerobic little Buddha brat, that is, if your mind is open to being reminded that the journey of saving a thousand neurons begins with taking a single step to restore all normal signaling, especially in the frontal lobe, so you are able to use your critical thinking skills so you can problem solve to your little heart's content.

'But first, Bratboy, you must free your mind of all prejudices neurologically associated with the fallacy of the perception aerobic exercise is simply a necessary evil and, instead, speak biochemical truth to the power of believing exercise is a necessary blessing.'

'LEAPING-LEGACY-OF-LABORATORY-LIZARDS, Bratman, what my brat-antennas are picking up is that a brat should get past the notion that exercise should be perceived as labor intensive and, instead, strive to enter into the promised land of an aerobic trancelike state of euphoria, for purposes of identification, hereinafter, known as Transylvania.'

'YES, brat-hopper, always remember, when it comes to helping to save brain cells by aerobically exercising, it is always better to have more mull and less whine.'

'HOLY-AEROBIC-HIGH-COVERS-A-MULTITUDE-OF-SYNAPSES, Bratman, I must know more of your promise of *cell-vation*!'

'WHOA, although your zeal is contagious, I feel I have a duty to warn children of the brat that unless they are willing to keep their neurological receiving coordinates locked on their frontal lobe, they somehow risk falling into the most notorious brat trap of all, which is exercising the belief that they are exercising by watching professional athletes run around on their big screen televisions.

'Unless a reasonable balance is struck, the ancient brat masters prophesied this primitive form of athletic couch *potatoism* as vicarious oxygenation or, as more modern legal brat scholars have put it, 'Sweat panting in the second part.'

'Holy-staying-sedentary-sitting-on-your-dairy-air, Bratman, all I know is there may be a loveable gullible couch potato out there, maybe even a spoiled little spud, yet one still yearning to know the aerobic truth, the whole aerobic truth, and nothing but the aerobic truth, and I will not rest until this small fry knows he has the cellular potential of becoming a world class *tater totter*.

'We must act now, now I tell you, Bratman, to save the children of the brat, who, if left to their own devices, will be left behind only to become accomplices to the ever expanding girth of a nation.

'To the brat mobile, Bratman, I say, to the brat mobile before my adrenaline rush dissipates and I am no longer able to use my self-righteous bratty indignation to expose children of the brat to the truth, to the light, to the new American aerobic way of helping to restore normal neuronal signaling so, together, we can band together to destroy the Otto Cratts of the world!!!'

'WHOA, calm down, calm down, Bratboy, inhale, while I take the time to blame myself for being a party to helping sell an overly simplistic dynamic dualistic superhero model of thinking.

'I mean, enough already with the light v. darkness thing or any other model, for that matter, which, I suspect, is the result of the brain processing indignation at the risk of our becoming self righteous.

'Admittedly, it's been a great marketing tool in promoting our own particular brat brand, but I am starting to realize this dynamic dualistic thinking model may not be all it's cracked up to be, especially if it means ignoring all the little demons lurking around in each of us with or without the help of Otto Cratt.'

'HOLY-SELF-REFLECTION, Bratman, let's postpone the idea of pillaging the countryside in the brat mobile in hopes of changing the lives of up and coming young brats until we have our own house in order.'

. . .

'HOW ABOUT, instead, we go for a drive and play your favorite brat road game Bratboy?'

'HOLY-SAY-IT-ISN'T-SO, Bratman, you don't mean, 'I spy with my little nuclei!'

'INDEED I DO. To the brat mobile!'

CHAPTER 16
JIMMY AND HIS HIGHNESS

"COUNSEL, let me pose a question. By first saying, you have attempted to make it abundantly clear throughout these proceedings that there are competing areas of the brain, which when a particular part is activated, that brain activity is expected to cause a certain effect, which when acted upon has consequences.

"And the Court can assume that the area of the brain we can freely associate with in order to initiate that particular chemical reaction will indeed, most likely, be influenced by the subjective experiences our brain cells have chosen to mirror.

"With that in mind, Counsel, my question is, is it your contention that those who have been diagnosed with Parkinson's still have time to choose a subjective experience which incorporates aerobic exercise into their lives, thereby giving them a fighting chance at keeping brain cells alive for a longer period of time?"

"WELL, your Honor, again, since everyone's personal experience with Parkinson's varies, it would depend greatly upon many factors and circumstances, including whether or not a person is still physically able to engage in aerobic exercise.

"With that exception, I agree with the Court's general description of my position. However, I would add that, depending on the reason or reasons why a brain cell is dying, the biochemical reaction made possible by inducing an aerobic high may help rather than can help to revive dying brain cells.

"But, for the record, I am willing to admit, there will be those diagnosed with Parkinson's, or who knowingly are at greater risk of having it, who may not be willing to make the necessary changes in their daily routine in order to lessen the disease."

"THE REASON BEING, COUNSEL?"

"BECAUSE THE CHOICE of neurologically tempering reason with motivation in order to engage in aerobic exercise is not yet an obvious first line of defense for some people."

"IT IS difficult for the Court to understand, Counsel, that those most at risk would do nothing other than take medications if they knew they had more control over their disease than they previously thought."

"WELL, your Honor, but I would, again, argue that only those who choose to gravitate toward activating the receptors in their rational brain are capable of engaging the critical thinking skills necessary to make decisions that lead to those important adjustments to their lifestyle."

"IS THERE a reasonable explanation as to why more rational receptors in the frontal lobe are not being used more often when important decisions are being made about health and well being, Counsel?"

"NOT TO MY KNOWLEDGE, your Honor, but perhaps at this stage of our evolution, we might still think that bouncing back and forth like a ping pong ball between the frontal lobe and different parts of the primordial brain is still the most effective way of surviving."

"INTERESTING, Counsel, but if science were able to more specifically define which groups posed a greater risk of being diagnosed with Parkinson's, the Court, using the reasonable person standard, would think that those in that particular population, in their own self interest to survive, would adopt a more pre-emptive aerobic lifestyle approach in order to have a fighting chance of staving off the disease."

"YOUR HONOR, the Court is to be praised for its optimism, but even when scientific studies continue to narrow the at-risk population in question, there does not seem to be a rush on gym memberships on the part of those in that particular demographic."

"CAN you point to one such recent study, Counsel?"

"WELL, your Honor, what recent scientific research has shown, at least in the case of a defective mitochondria (oven), is that such a defect can lead to a mitochondrial DNA disease, of which Parkinson's is one.

178

"Indeed, what scientists have concluded is that mito-chondrial DNA is inherited without any of the father's sperm, which means mitochondrial DNA diseases, like Parkinson's disease, are only capable of being passed along from mother to child. (Reference, *Powering the Brain: An Introduction to Mitochondria,*" by Professor Doug Turnbull, Think Neuroscience, January 16, 2013.)"

"SO, Counsel, what you are saying is that there is already a suspect classification of those who may be at a greater risk for getting Parkinson's, and that can be de-termined by examining whether a maternal line can be indicated for having had a history of the disease, at least as far as having gotten the disease resulted from having defective mitochondria."

"YES, your Honor, at least insofar as mitochondrial disease induced Parkinson's is concerned, that is, if that particular study is assumed to be correct."

"COUNSEL, why don't we change directions by now having you give the Court some historical background to help us put Parkinson's disease into better context?"

. . .

"OF COURSE, your Honor, when the disease is put into a historical context, the evidence will show that if Dr. James Parkinson (1755-1824), hereinafter referred to as 'Jimmy' (pronounced gym-eey), were alive today, he would be getting closer to being able to blow out three hundred candles on his birthday cake."

"COUNSEL, how has the treatment of the disease evolved after nearly three hundred years?"

"WELL, your Honor, I would say, over the centuries, the science has evolved to the point where it has relied, as the evidence has shown, almost exclusively on a medication targeting method model, which, in other words, brings something outside the brain into the brain, i.e., a drug, which is designed to find its way across the blood brain barrier to a very specific place inside the brain in order to replace or replicate a once active byproduct (dopamine) of a dead brain cell that, when in its prime, functioned by helping us to move about more freely.

"Science, arguably, until recently, has not made a big deal about our doing something inside the brain on our own, like igniting a chemical reaction by exercising as a way of setting in motion a daily deep brain stimulation of brain cells."

. . .

"SO, Counsel, what it seems you are implying is that there is little chance of finding a cure so long as medical science stays on the same path it has been on for centuries."

"WELL, your Honor, never say never, but, yes, it is my position that modern medicine will be spinning its wheels if it continues down the same path it is on instead of changing its focus."

"WHICH FOCUS WOULD THAT BE?"

"AGAIN, in my humble opinion, by figuring out a way of keeping brain cells alive."

"DR. JAMES PARKINSON discovered the disease; in what year, Counsel?"

"1817, YOUR HONOR."

. . .

"SO, Counsel, is it fair to assume that after having first discovered the disease, Dr. Parkinson made no attempts at finding a cure?"

"NOT TO MY KNOWLEDGE, but in defense of Jimmy, your Honor, his instincts were actually quite revelatory when you considered that he suggested that taking drugs to treat the disease was, at that time, not indicated, when he wrote, 'Until we are better informed respecting the nature of the disease, the employment of internal medicines is scarcely warranted; unless analogy should point out some remedy the trial of which rational hope might authorize.' (Citation, Parkinson's, James, *Essay on the Shaking Palsy*, London: Whittingham and Rowland, 1817, p. 62)."

"BUT TO BE FAIR, he neither recommended aerobic exercise as a way of treating what he called *shaking palsy*, Counsel."

"NO, but let me remind the Court that in the day of Jimmy, without having had the benefit of magnetic resonance imaging (MRI) to be able to appreciate the fact each brain cell is a separate structural unit, let alone knowing each neuron came custom made with its own power station (mitochondria), it would have been nearly impossible for him to make the connection between aerobic exercise and keeping brain cells alive to fight Parkinson's, all related dementias for that matter, and the remarkably predictable outcome of depression inherent with the death of brain cells, especially the ones that regulate the use of serotonin, acetylcholine, or dopamine (SAD).

"But if he had been able to make this connection, your Honor, and if by some silly twist of fate, Jimmy, let's say, rather than being a London surgeon, had become the first sports medicine doctor, and let's throw into the hypothetical, he had had the royal ear of the King of England, George III (1738-1820), then he, Jimmy, may have been able to change the course of history by convincing His Highness to convert a wing in the palace into a gym where he could induce a runner's high every day."

"AND WHY WOULD this be relevant, Counsel, in the case of George III?"

"YOUR HONOR, a home gym would have given King George a place where he would have been able to condition himself to where His Highness would be able to induce the highest of most royal aerobic highs, which may have had the added benefit of helping to curb his depression, which a palatial nurse observed and described as being 'melancholy beyond description.' (Citation, Hibbert, Christopher, *George III: A Personal History,* London: Penguin Books, 1999, p. 394.)"

"COUNSEL, YOUR POINT, PLEASE."

"YOUR HONOR, my hypothetical shows that whether a person is born a prince or a pauper, evolution has been very democratic in the way it has given each of us the ability to use reason to find out the neurological benefits of defending and protecting the constitution of brain cells by being able to enjoy the same benefits of inducing a runner's *highness.*"

"WELL, Counsel, the Court thinks it is high time you move on to another subject."

"BY ALL MEANS, YOUR HONOR."

CHAPTER 17

GOOD COPER, BAD COPER

"SO, Counsel, the evidence again seems to suggest the wheels of aerobic justice turn slowly, that is, if they turn at all."

"YES, your Honor, but in defense of the modern medical trend, the brain health value of intense aerobic exercise, particularly for those in the early stages of Parkinson's disease, is beginning to gain traction." (Citations, Fitzgerald, Susan, *Early PD Patients May Benefit from Exercising at a High Intensity,* Neurology Today, January 25, 2018, p.20; and Reynolds, Gretchen, *Exercise May Aid Parkinson's Disease, but Make It Intense,* The New York Times, Dec. 13, 2017).

. . .

"STILL, Counsel, there does not yet seem to be a groundswell amongst those in the medical community who are willing to put diet and exercise on the same level of importance as taking drugs to curb symptoms."

"YOUR HONOR, as far as I know, aerobic exercise is not yet a staple in any medical school curriculum, but the evidence, again, clearly shows that the scientific literature is beginning to connect the dots between exercise and brain health."

"ARE you ready to offer into evidence any such learned treatises on the subject at this time?"

"I AM, your Honor, if the Court deems it appropriate."

"YES, it so deems, but in the interests of judicial economy, Counsel, the Court would ask you to limit your response to just a sampling."

"WELL THEN, your Honor, for the Court's consideration, I would offer the following:

"First, there is *Navigating Life with Parkinson Disease* (New York: Oxford University Press, 2013, p. 191), where Sotirios A. Parashos, MD, PhD, explains, 'Exercise is recommended as part of a fully integrated treatment program for people with Parkinson's. The benefits of exercise are many and include improved strength, bone health, flexibility, and endurance. Recent studies suggest that exercise may have a disease-modifying effect on helping remaining dopamine cells to function more efficiently.'

"Then there is *Training Your Brain for Dummies* (West Sussex: A. John Wiley and Sons, Ltd. Publication, 2011, p. 158), where Tracy Pacoima Dalloway, PhD, Director of the Center for Memory in the Lifespan at the University of Sterling, UK, gives details on how 'studies have confirmed that aerobic activity leads to more benefits for your brain than activities that focus on concentration and toning... As people grow older, the human brain begins to lose tissue, which results in the deterioration of cognitive skills. Aerobic exercise is one clear way to delay and in some cases even reverse the effects that age and injury have on the brain.'

"Thirdly, in *Magnificent Mind at Any Age* (New York: Harmony Books, 2008, p. 28), Daniel G. Amen, M.D., puts it in plain words, 'The brain needs physical exercise. Without it, the brain struggles. Exercise boosts blood flow to the brain, which helps supply oxygen, glucose, and nutrients and takes away toxic substances...if the deep areas of the brain are starved of healthy blood flow you will have problems with coordination and processing complex thoughts.'

"And, your Honor, what may be more on point with regard to these proceedings, *The Brain's Way of Healing,* (New York: Viking Press, 2015, p. 83). Norman Doidge, M.D., elucidates, 'It was found that the dopamine-producing system in the substantia nigra had been better preserved in the animals that exercised... Another major breakthrough has been the finding that when Parkinson's-like animals exercise, they produce two kinds of growth factors: GDNF (glial-derived neurotrophic factor) and BDNF (brain-derived neurotrophic factor) in their brains that permits them to form new connections between brain cells.'

"One source already mentioned, but bears repeating, is *Spark, The Revolutionary New Science of Exercise and the Brain* (New York: Little Brown and Company, 2008, p. 135), where John J. Ratey, M.D., points out, '... exercise doesn't selectively influence anything—it adjusts the chemistry of the entire brain to restore normal signaling.'

"Another work I would add is *Future Bright, A Transforming Vision of Human Intelligence* (New York Oxford University Press, 2013, p. 248), where Michael E. Martinez, PhD, adds, 'For reasons that are still being elucidated, exercise stimulates the brain to create new structures that are fundamental to its effective operation. Structural improvements occur in two forms---more extensive vascularization and a greater number of synapses that connect neurons.'"

"COUNSEL, would you like to offer any other scientific documentation into evidence at this time?"

"NOT AT THIS TIME, your Honor, but I would like to take a moment for the Court to sit in amazement at how two of the ideas just cited, i.e., '...the dopamine-producing system in the substantia nigra had been better preserved in the animals that exercised' (Doidge, p. 83) and '...exercise adjusts the chemistry of the entire brain to restore normal signaling' (Ratey, p. 135). These two have just found their way to each other through time and space to make their way into this courtroom in order to lend credence to the integrity of my main argument."

"CONSIDER THE COURT AMAZED, Counsel, but, again, to be clear, you are not suggesting those with Parkinson's disease stop taking medications, no matter whether they rely upon high intensity aerobic therapy or not."

. . .

"THAT'S CORRECT, your Honor, and again, they would be well advised to get their doctor's approval before choosing an aerobic coping strategy, regardless of whether this strategy is done with or without the use of prescription medications."

"WITH THAT SAID, Counsel, what were your first impressions when you began using aerobic therapy as a way of treating your Parkinson's disease?"

"WELL, your Honor, from the moment I began to use an elliptical machine, I noticed that the tremor in my right hand would stop, at least while I was on the machine.

"From the onset, then, it became very clear to me that treating a movement disorder with movement was having a positive effect."

"HOW DID you come to believe that movement was having a positive effect?"

. . .

"YOUR HONOR, it has, in part, to do with the understanding that compromised body parts afflicted by the disease, e.g., legs and limbs, are probably less mobile and thus no longer able to send decipherable electrical signals vibrant enough to receptors in that part of the brain to which they, the compromised parts, are directly connected.

"And, in my opinion, when those evolutionary designed motion detectors, i.e., receptors in the brain, linked to those particular afflicted body parts are left unstimulated, brain cells that otherwise would be called into action probably just die for want of having the motion necessary to stay alive.

"In other words, your Honor, what I believe happens when people use, let's say, an elliptical machine, unlike a treadmill or stationary bike, is that they engage their arms in particular in a repetitive motion, arms that otherwise would probably remain dormant, which, in turn, has the effect of sending critical signals to the applicable receptors in the brain to which those body parts are connected.

"And when said receptors in the brain receive said signals, the resulting electrically charged activity gives those particular neurons the incentive they need to send out movement information back to the body parts being targeted, arms and legs, and that simple act of stimulation, I would argue, helps to keep those particular brain cells alive." (Reference, *Leg Exercise is Critical to Brain and Nervous System Health,* Frontiers in Neuroscience, as reported in SCIENMAG, Science Magazine.)

"FOR THE RECORD, Counsel, how did you end up choosing an elliptical as your exercise machine of choice to battle Parkinson's?"

"YOUR HONOR, I often used an elliptical machine to deal with the stress of being a lawyer, especially when I was getting ready for a trial.

"So after having been diagnosed with Parkinson's and facing a new brand of stress to the point where my self-image was at risk, I found solace getting back on an elliptical machine, which I saw as an old friend."

"COUNSEL, you say your self-image was sinking?"

"YES, your Honor, my self-image had sunk so low that not even a cyber-thief was interested in stealing my identity."

. . .

"THAT'S PRETTY DARN LOW, Counsel, but, then you say, a seminal moment occurred while on an elliptical machine, where you allege your tremor stopped as long as you continued using the machine?"

"YES, your Honor, I repeated the experience the next day and, schedule permitting, every day since."

"CAN you explain what it was about using the machine that kept you coming back?"

"WELL, your Honor, having been a distance runner in the day, my dream has been to harken back to the much coveted runner's high I was able to trigger as a youth.

"Not until I was diagnosed with Parkinson's did I realize how easy it would be to come close to fulfilling that dream by using this joint-friendly technology."

"AS AN ASIDE, are you representing to the Court you were once some sort of elite athlete, Counsel?"

. . .

"NOT HARDLY, your Honor, but I will say, the older I get, the better athlete I was."

"COUNSEL, that is common among most of us; please continue."

"SO, on my quest to resurrect the alleged glory days by using an elliptical machine, your Honor, serendipitously, I came to discover that the closer and closer I came to fulfilling my dream of inducing the coveted runner's high, the longer and longer the period of time that would elapse between my tremors.

"Indeed, over time, what I came to ascertain was that there seemed to be a correlation between sullying symptoms for a day or two and triggering a sense of well being, like I once felt when getting a runner's high."

"AND YOU THINK your experience could be replicated in the brains of others similarly situated as you, Counsel?"

"YOUR HONOR, I will admit to the Court, I would be on very thin ice thinking my experience could be replicated in most others with Parkinson's, because every person's disease is so different, and besides, I would find it necessary to warn people of the addiction created by relying on daily aerobic exercise.

"Let's say, in other words, that if a person makes an aerobic choice and the choice happens to work for him or her, it should also be disclosed that what is probably being done, with the best of intentions, is the creation of a self-imposed chemical dependency that comes with trying to create a daily runner's high."

"STILL, Counsel, the Court would consider this to be a healthy addiction, as most addictions are so long as the reward system stays connected and closely supervised, as you have argued, with the prefrontal cortex."

"PERHAPS, but for the sake of transparency, a person should be made aware, if he or she chooses aerobic therapy and diet as his or her coping mechanisms of choice, there may evolve a healthy craving for a daily fix.

"So just saying, your Honor, under the heading of 'forewarned is forearmed,' if one becomes a Parkinson's purist, so to speak, by choosing to cope with the disease by attempting, aerobically, to induce a chemical high every day in order to restore normal neuronal signaling (good coper), but then suddenly stops without just cause (bad coper), this person should be made aware there is the risk of suffering a withdrawal when brain cells are put on notice they are no longer first party beneficiaries to a 'healthy' addiction."

"NONETHELESS, Counsel, assuming hypothetically, there are class of citizens willing to remain loyal to an aerobic cause and effect because that works for them, that should be their choice, especially if it means they are able to bring a dying brain cell back to some semblance of life, now let's move on."

CHAPTER 18

MOTION AS MEDICINE

"WHAT SHOULD ALSO BE ADDED to the record, your Honor, when I opted for using elliptically induced motion as medicine, it took weeks of conditioning before I was able to reach a certain point of being fit enough to be able to generate the threshold amount of electro-chemical energy necessary to induce the coveted runner's high and, thereby, restore relative normal signaling to the brain."

"AND YOU, Counsel, would have the Court believe you were able to do this chemical charging of your brain by using an elliptical machine."

. . .

"YES, your Honor, but I would hasten to add, again, that what has worked for me may not work for others, so I must caution..."

"NO MORE 'BUTS' allowed into evidence Counsel, you have made it abundantly clear to the Court you don't want to disappoint anyone, but I can assure you from what the Court has heard so far, it has a reasonable expectation, only a handful of those willing to read this transcript will attempt to replicate your daily exercise routine."

"NO OFFENSE TAKEN, but I would ask for a finding from the Court as to why it thinks so few people reading this transcript will use motion as a way of coping with their movement disorder."

"WELL, Counsel, if I may comment on the evidence as it has been presented so far, in order for a neuron to inculcate a learned behavior, a neuron needs a frame of reference, something to mirror, in order for it to mimic something else, such as exercise.

"The Court is therefore willing to make an initial finding that a brain cell is likely to mimic only what it sees and, therefore, will act only upon what a person has stored up in his or her memory bank as a unique repertoire of subjective experiences.

"And in our culture, since motion has not yet been inculcated into the collective consciousness as medicine, it has little if any chance of being used by a majority of people as a way of coping with their disease, certainly not with the same enthusiasm as prescription medications.

"Thus, if no meaningful aerobic exercise protocol had ever been stored in its modeling memory of the collective consciousness, neurons could not be expected to arise en masse and be willing, on their own, neurologically speaking, to anchor to something as foreign as thinking exercise should be taken as seriously as taking medications to control something as formidable as the symptoms of a progressive brain disease.

"Counsel, it's nothing personal, and that is not to say you cannot win an occasional case of first impression with someone here or there who may be straddling the aerobic option fence.

"So please, for that select group of people, continue by sharing what it is about using an elliptical machine that has its advantages for them."

. . .

"WELL, what I discovered using an elliptical machine, your Honor, is that since there is no pounding motion, it is relatively stress-free on the joints, which reduces the risk of repetitive stress injuries."

"COUNSEL, are elliptical machines as joint friendly as, say, a treadmill?"

"MORE FRIENDLY, but quite frankly, your Honor, I try to avoid any exercise equipment or running where there is any pounding whatsoever, believing, as go the knees, so goes the 'cure'.

"More specifically, there is another more general concern I have about treadmills where they may pose a higher degree of risk of injury if, let's say, a Parkinson's patient gets dizzy or feels faint and is not able to stop the treadmill, he or she might end up as a wall hanging because the machine does not slow down on its own, whereas an elliptical machine slows down when the user slows down and stops moving.

"This may explain why it is estimated that accidents on treadmills cause about 24,000 injuries annually amongst the general population." (Citation, Bachman, Rachel, *Treadmills Unplugged: A Workout Powered by Your Feet*, The Wall Street Journal, July 7, 2015, p. D1.)

. . .

"AGAIN, Counsel, just so we are clear, explain why you do not have the same concerns about this happening while you are on an elliptical machine."

"SO, your Honor, assuming hypothetically, I get dizzy on an elliptical machine, I have control over the motion being generated simply by stopping my own movement, which is causing the machine to move.

"But even with that advantage, I would still caution a beginner using an elliptical machine; it, no doubt, will initially create in him or her a sense of being uncoordinated until that part of the brain, the cerebellum, kicks in and has had a chance to inculcate new learned skilled motor movements.

"Over time, when a person graduates to the level of joining the ranks of the elliptical elite, he or she might even have the confidence of reversing the direction of the movement, which at first can cause a sense of being uncoordinated, until, again, the cerebellum has a chance to work its magic inculcating even more newly learned skilled motor movements to boot and reboot.

"So until the cerebellum kicks in with its new learned motor movement that allows a person to exercise at an accelerated level, in an abundance of caution, it might be helpful to have someone, maybe a personal trainer, a friend, or a family member, spot the user until he or she gets his or her elliptical legs, so to speak."

"COUNSEL, could you refresh the Court's memory as to the function of the cerebellum?"

"YES, your Honor, if my notes are correct, I think Dr. Marx said something to the effect that the cerebellum, home to about half of our brain cells, is found at the base of the brain and controls coordination of voluntary movement, gross and fine motor skills, posture, and balance; indeed, it is a learned skilled motor movement machine, cranking out more movement pathways than, he said, a well landscaped and architecturally friendly retirement community.

"And he also pointed out that it is important for us to know about the insatiable appetite the cerebellum has for refining movement, let's say by getting on an elliptical machine and trying to move arms and legs simultaneously while factoring in the survival instinct of not falling or losing balance."

. . .

"COUNSEL, is there anything else you have to add regarding your use of an elliptical machine?"

"WELL, yes, your Honor, I have also found that while using an elliptical, I am able to keep my eyes closed, and I have found this to be an important part of my exercise regimen and would therefore ask the Court to allow me to explain."

"COUNSEL, since the very act of keeping your eyes closed would prohibit the safe use of most exercise equipment, save, perhaps, an elliptical machine or stationary bicycle, the Court will not only indulge you, but it will also insist you make an offer of proof."

"SO, your Honor, it's purely theoretical on my part, but I believe that by keeping my eyes closed while safely enjoying the movement of an elliptical machine, I am making an effort to shut off other competing areas of the brain that might otherwise be competing for electro-chemical stimulation, i.e., other competing areas of the brain and all that stuff.

"This way I can focus all my attention on the miracle of movement in an attempt to understand what is really going on in the brain on a microscopic level."

"AND YOU THINK this helps target more electrochemical activity in the compromised part of your brain that causes you to have Parkinson's disease."

"YES, your Honor, the substantia nigra in the basal ganglia."

"DO YOU KNOW, Counsel, which competing parts cause the greatest distractions for most people?"

"WELL, your Honor, again, this is speculative on my part, but it would only make sense that by keeping my eyes closed, I am attempting to shut out all visual distractions, which would trigger a chemical reaction in the occipital lobe, which in turn would trigger chemical reactions in other competing areas of the brain for purposes of assessing what has been seen."

. . .

"CAN YOU GIVE ME AN EXAMPLE, Counsel, of a visual distraction setting in motion competing areas of the brain?"

"WELL, your Honor, the most obvious visual distraction while on the elliptical machine is the ever-present television, which depending on what we choose to watch, can further cause to activate other competing areas of the brain, for example, an emotion in our limbic system or a fear in the amygdala.

"The only point I am trying to make, your Honor, is that if a person with Parkinson's disease truly believes that trying to induce an aerobic high has the capacity of restoring normal signaling in remaining brain cells, then in order to get the best bang for his or her exercise buck, a person may be at a disadvantage from the start by wasting mental energy on reality television or the constant stream of breaking news rather than by going into a trancelike state, with eyes closed, and becoming immersed in the healing energy that can only be found within."

"POINT TAKEN, Counsel; now let's move on."

. . .

"YOUR HONOR, before resting my case and proceeding with my closing argument, I would ask for the Court's guidance on how it wants to proceed."

"THANK YOU, COUNSEL."

CHAPTER 19
LOOSE ENDS

"COUNSEL, before I allow you to give your summation, for the record, I need clarification on certain issues, including whether *Lewy bodies*, whose accumulation you claim can be one of the proximate causes of Parkinson's disease, can negatively affect other parts of the brain as well."

"YES, your Honor, so Lewy Body Dementia (LBD) is actually a brain disease in and of itself and, again, is associated with abnormal deposits of alpha-synuclein, a protein that can be lethal when clumped together in the frontotemporal part of the brain.

"These *Lewy bodies* deposits can affect thinking, movement, behavior, and mood, and LBD can occur alone or along with a progressive brain disease like Parkinson's." (Reference, National Institute of Health, NIH Publication No. 13-7907, 2013, p. 2.)

"But when *Lewy bodies* invade higher cognitive functioning parts of the brain, it is no longer called Parkinson's, but LBD, named after Dr. Frederick Lewy (1885-1950), a neurologist who, ironically, first discovered these blobs of defective protein (again, synuclein) in the neurons in that part of the basal ganglia called the *substantia nigra*, again, relevant in Parkinson's disease."

"THANK YOU; another loose end, Counsel, has to do with explaining the differences, if any, between a progressive brain disease and a brain injury resulting from an accident or athletic endeavor."

"IN LIGHT of my own trial experience, your Honor, most of my brain injury litigation resulted from blunt head traumas that caused what is known as axonal shearing.

"Most injuries were what expert witnesses often referred to as coup, contra-coup type injuries, which happen when the head is hit so hard that the brain, which is often compared to Jell-O, bounces around, often striking sharp parts of the front and back of the skull's surfaces, causing serious injuries if enough brain cells are destroyed.

"One difference between people with Parkinson's disease and people with blunt head trauma is that people with blunt head trauma are more likely to have a shearing effect on the axons of their brain cells, which is caused by the rapid acceleration and deceleration of the brain during trauma.

"Shearing in enough neurons can cause a permanent impairment of the nucleus (a cluster of brain cells with specific functions) unless the brain restores function by re-circuiting neuropathways, often referred to as brain plasticity, the rerouting of which can also occur when a person engages in vigorous aerobic exercise.

"Another difference between head injuries and brain disease is that in head trauma cases, radiological studies would often show lesions causing impairment, usually in one of the four lobes (frontal, temporal, parietal, or occipital), with each respective lobe responsible for controlling specific brain functions.

"For example, a lesion or injury to the frontal lobe might result in difficulty with, among other things, problem solving or executive decision making; a lesion(s) or injury to the temporal lobe might result in, among other things, a loss of short term memory or language comprehension; a lesion(s) or injury to the parietal lobe might result in, among other things, problems with spatial orientation or hand-eye coordination; and a lesion(s) or injury to the occipital lobe might result in, usually, some type of visual impairment.

"Your Honor, I might add that if multiple lesions were found in more than one part of the brain, I would try to convince the jury that my client did not have a brain injury, but rather multiple brain injuries, each of which permanently changed the structure of one of the only known organisms in the universe that knows it exists.

"When everything is taken into consideration, however, what a progressive brain disease and brain injuries do have in common is that in each, neurons no longer exist as they once did and therefore are no longer able to function as they were intended to function, which changes a person forever.

"In other words, in both cases, everything points to the fact that brain cells have lost their ability, due to a lack of plasticity, to have an electrochemically charged relationship with nearby neurons. This means that they can't pass on important information like how to move, think, learn, and remember.

"The insidious thing about head trauma is that when faced with being bluntly struck, there is usually no warning, allowing a person the opportunity to take evasive action.

"On the other hand, the silver lining as far as progressive brain diseases are concerned is that in their early stages there are usually many early warning signals, giving a person the option to be proactive in attempting to control the behavior, and thus the momentum, of the disease.

"The good news is that the early onset of Parkinson's symptoms, which may cause a Parkinson's panic that keeps us stuck in our fear center (the amygdala), will, when cooler, more rational parts of the brain take over, be understood to mean that we might benefit a lot by just making some changes to our lifestyle."

"NEXT, Counsel, I thought it might be helpful for us to understand how long it has taken humanity to discover brain cells are separate units and why that is important."

"JUST TO GIVE it some historical context, your Honor, while the higher functioning parts of our brain in the cerebral cortex have been busy evolving for, let's say, two million years, it has only been within the last hundred years or so that we have come to discover a brain cell is a separate structural unit.

"This critical bit of information, that a brain cell is a separate structural unit, was the result of research done by

Santiago Ramon y Cajol (1852-1934), not to be con-fused with another theory being shopped around the same time in the early part of the last century, which was that the neuro-system was not made up of separate units but by some kind of elaborate neuronet, an idea being peddled by Camillo Golgi (1843-1926).

"This notion that a neuron is a separate unit must not yet have been accepted science in 1906 since both scholars, Professors Cajol and Golgi, had to share the Nobel Prize.

"The scuttlebutt in the halls of science was that even though they did share the Nobel Prize, they did so reluc-tantly, each holding firmly to their respective net and no-net theories.

"Apparently, your Honor, this particular breed of scien-tists, although not known for being particularly militant, apparently could still get quite testy at that time when the two theories were being hotly contested, which may have created a great deal of science friction."

"DON'T GO DOWN that path, Counsel; we'll have no more of that."

. . .

"SORRY, your Honor. Getting back to your question and emphasizing just how recently we learned that a brain cell was a separate structural unit, it might help to see where said discovery fits on a timeline based upon approximately how long we have been using our rational brain.

"If two million years of cerebral cortex evolution and its development represented exactly one mile, one hundred years, since discovering a neuron is a separate structural unit, would represent less than .03 inch of that mile, and the discovery of Parkinson's would represent less than .05 inch of that mile.

"With this in mind, it is worth noting that while the cerebral cortex, for two million years, had been getting all smart and stuff, the basal ganglia, where Parkinson's disease originates, apparently was quite satisfied with having evolved as much as it was going to evolve up until that time, that is, when the rational brain was just starting to take its evolution more seriously."

"WHY DO you think it is relevant that we understand a brain cell to be understood as a separate structural unit, Counsel?"

. . .

"WHAT IT SAYS TO ME, your Honor, is that if each brain cell is an island unto itself, vastly interconnected electrically with other islands, that absent this biochemical electrical activity, the neuron will no longer think its structural integrity is necessary in the grand scheme of things and, thus, risks becoming obsolete when there is minimal movement.

"But what is important to know in light of these proceedings is that by forcing the brain cells to feel the effects of vigorous aerobic activity, especially on the ones connected to certain compromised body parts, arms and legs, this may be all the stimulation necessary to keep these particular brain cells fully functioning for the time being."

"COUNSEL, just so there is absolutely no confusion, it might help if you were to remind the Court, again, of the part of the brain that is implicated in Parkinson's disease."

"I WILL TOUCH upon that more in detail in my closing argument, your Honor, but, to review, what the evidence has shown is that people with Parkinson's disease have brain cells in their substantial nigra, located in the basal ganglia, that mature prematurely, and, thus, dopamine, a neurotransmitter, does not get produced and projected out into the muscles at amounts necessary to assure normal movement.

"I might add, our distant nomadic ancestors (based on our DNA) probably relied more on their basal ganglia for their survival than we might ever imagine.

"Indeed, being able to move with reliable coordination and being more cunning than a saber tooth tiger, or anything with sharper teeth for that matter, would ultimately determine who would have whom for lunch."

"YOUR POINT, COUNSEL?"

"THE POINT IS, your Honor, at the time it was being decided whether the prehistoric menu would offer a cave crepe or a saber tooth soufflé, our DNA probably had more electrochemical dopamine charged inputs than a caveman could shake a stick or a club at.

"And he could remember where he stuck that stick because he was, all the while, passing information from one brain cell to another brain cell in yet another old area of the brain, the hippocampus, where memory is stored and retrieved in emergency situations that may have necessitated a quick response."

. . .

"IT SOUNDS, Counsel, as if necessity is the mother of invention, then survival is the offspring of being able to move."

"YES, your Honor, for those with Parkinson's and related progressive brain diseases, one would think there would be more than a passing interest in knowing the exact point in time when survival and movement were no longer the Fred Astaire and Ginger Rogers of evolution.

"Indeed, my suspicion is that when the reptilian brain, more specifically for our purposes, the brainstem, began to sense movement, it was no longer a critical instinctual component of our immediate survival, and I think we have to at least ask the question whether we became more vulnerable to movement disorders since those particular brain cells were, by default, no longer the focus of being electrically stimulated."

"SO WHAT YOU'RE SAYING, Counsel, is that the less we needed to move in order to survive had unintended consequences on the brain."

. . .

"WHY YES, your Honor, if, indeed, some type of brainstem devolution is going on, resulting in less movement, the eternal optimist in me is willing to concede that even if our species is in the early stages of losing its ability to move as fluidly as our DNA, it still has had a fantastic run.

"When you begin to peel the onion, your Honor, we have gone from cave dwellers to hunter gatherer, to herders, to farmers, to fishermen, to industrial workers, to salespeople, to computer scientists, and, finally, after two million years, we have crossed the finish line by choosing to be couch potatoes."

"IF WHAT YOU say is true, Counsel, how did we end up in this sluggish place?"

"NO ONE CAN SAY with scientific certainty, your Honor, but what deserves close scrutiny is looking at what was happening industrially at or near the time when James Parkinson was born on April 11, 1755.

"That cute little bouncing baby boy saw the first light of day on the eve of the Industrial Revolution, and by the time he was all grown up and discovered somebody shaking like a leaf in a windstorm, in 1817, the Industrial Revolution was already in full swing."

. . .

"SO THE ISSUE you are posing, Counsel, is what part, if any, did the Industrial Revolution play, externally, in being yet another proximate cause?"

"WELL, yes, but an alert defense attorney would point out, your Honor, except for early onset, for the most part, Parkinson's is an older person's disease, and most people were not living as long prior to the Industrial Revolution to be able to get it in the first place, and besides, he or she would also be able to correctly point out, Parkinson's symptoms were recorded in India and China thousands of years ago."

"HOW WOULD YOU RESPOND, COUNSEL?"

"TO WHICH I WOULD RESPOND, true, less longevity was probably a factor, but amongst the population of people who did live longer, e.g., the landed gentry and royalty, there still did not seem to be a lot of reported cases.

"And as far as reported cases going way back, that is also probably true, but there is not a sense of the same magnitude of diagnosed cases being cranked out, e.g., 90,000 a year in the United States alone, and rising faster than what feels reasonable."

"DO you notice any similarities between Parkinson's disease, Counsel, and any other global crisis we are facing today?"

"WELL, your Honor, Parkinson's disease, I suppose, is similar to global warming in that we have always had hurricanes, tsunamis, and tornadoes, just as we probably have always had Parkinson's, but the relevant question is not whether or not these natural disasters have or have not always existed, but rather whether they are becoming more severe.

"With regards to Parkinson's disease, the most obvious related issue is what, if any, effect post industrial chemicals have had on our neurons, e.g., pesticides, herbicides, weed killers, bug sprays, over five hundred chemicals used in fracking (some of which are considered proprietary and therefore not disclosed, legislated as the Halliburton exception), fertilizers, white phosphorous, depleted uranium, plutonium, carbon, and radiation emissions, to name a few of the usual suspects."

. . .

"COUNSEL, is there anything you would like to add before I ask you to make your closing argument?"

"WELL, your Honor, parenthetically, I should also mention something that may be perceived as a collateral matter but is arguably just as harmful as chemical toxins, and that is the role the industrial revolution may, unwittingly, have played in the creation of the No-Movement Movement.

"Since the industrial revolution, as already suggested, we have slowly drifted toward the couch potato era, where our favorite form of exercise is to watch professional athletes exercise."

"COUNSEL, it would seem that in order for a person to adapt to a lifestyle change, like getting off the couch to exercise, there would appear to be a need to self-reflect."

"YOUR HONOR, the discomfort of self-reflection can go deep and usually on a cellular level. It is commensurate with how much synaptic cement was laid by earlier subjective experiences that created the later need for self-reflection in the first place.

"Each time, for example, we might even choose to validate a bad feeling about exercise because we, subconsciously, may associate it, let's say, with having had a bad exercise experience."

"THANK YOU, Counsel. Any final words before you close?"

"SO, your Honor, I would just like to emphasize the importance of understanding the critical objective of keeping brain cells alive, so we might be able to move about more freely and think more clearly, and that we hold the key to our own neuronal cell by becoming more aware we have the power to create an electro-chemical reaction, able to unlock the vitality of brain cells throughout the entire brain with diet and exercise."

"COUNSEL, are you prepared to give your closing argument?"

"YES, YOUR HONOR."

CHAPTER 20
CLOSING ARGUMENT

"IT WAS ONCE SAID that we become what we think about, but what the evidence has revealed in these proceedings is that what we decide to think about is greatly influenced by which area of the brain we choose to activate in order to process the thought, which ultimately determines who we become, which, in turn, greatly influences the actions we take.

"Along those same lines, when it was said that we don't see the world as it is, but rather as we are, it is also important to note the evidence has also shown this is because the world we see is seen through a lens constructed by the sum total of our subjective experiences.

"In our quest to understand truths that are self-evident, it was shown that there exists within each of us civilizations of brain cells that have evolved into separate structural units, each of which, depending upon the task, is designed in a way that was configured to pass vital information between neurons primarily during most of our existence as the primary way in which we have survived.

"To this end, the evidence began by showing that even though each neuron is a separate structural unit, each brain cell identifies itself with a particular nucleus, which, I suggested, could be thought of as a band of like-minded brain cells, the purpose or function of which depends upon the area of the brain to which it has evolved.

"For purposes of clarification, I attempted to liken a nucleus to a street gang made up of like minded gang members (brain cells), who, again, have evolved to a specific area of the brain turf because they (brain cells) share the same territorial function.

"It was further shown that everything works well so long as electrically signaled information is able to pass unencumbered between like minded brain cells.

"But since the cellular universe within each of us, like the real world outside of us, is not perfect, we learned that communication between brain cells can sometimes break down when information between neurons becomes impossible to electrochemically pass between each other because of excess amounts of protein, which led to the notion of 'gunk science'.

"It was, therefore, shown that gang members (brain cells) get gunked and risk death when there becomes too much protein or filaments; there is no threat if normal in the right amounts, but excess can gum up or gunk the inner workings of a brain cell, preventing information from being passed.

"A presentation was made to the Court of an example of the dire consequences that can occur when there are excessive amounts of a particular protein in brain cells called *Lewy bodies*, which, when harvested excessively in a certain part of the basal ganglia (substantia nigra), can become one of the many proximate causes of Parkinson's disease.

"Next, when the Court became curious as to how information was passed between brain cells, it was first explained how the space between brain cells is called the synapse and how chemical information is carried across this synapse via neurotransmitters and how said chemical interacts with receptors on the postsynaptic membrane of another brain cell.

"One neurotransmitter in particular, called dopamine, was highlighted because its shortage is directly related to the death of brain cells, which can cause the symptoms we experience in Parkinson's disease.

"It was also noteworthy to point out that dopamine is either excitatory or inhibitory, suggesting its neuro-transmitting key capacity was designed by evolution to be able to unlock at least two different types of postsy-naptic receptors depending upon whether or not it is appropriate to move.

"An action potential is decided in a place within the neuron called the axon hillock.

"So there would be no confusion about what informa-tion meant in a cellular context, it was explained to the Court that the passing between neurons is not just about passing knowledge or thought as we typically think about knowledge or thought having to do with memory, emotion, or learning (MEL) in the limbic system.

"But a more expansive definition of how information passes between brain cells when we do things like breathing, sleeping, and heart-beating, a function of the brain stem.

"Or more to the point of these proceedings, the passing between brain cells of movement information as done in the primary motor cortex, premotor cortex, cerebellum (coordination), pyramidal motor system, and extrapyra-midal motor system.

"At that particular point in the proceedings, I thought it would be helpful, in order to come to a better overall understanding of a neuron, to concentrate not only on what goes on inside a brain cell, but to focus our attention on activities outside the neuron as well.

"To that end, the function of an astrocyte was introduced into evidence, something referred to as a glial cell, a star shaped support cell surrounding a neuron, evolutionarily charged to be (cells) body guards, designed to protect them from toxic waste, provide them with nutrients, keep them insulated, and, more recently, thought to play an important role in memory and sleep.

"By turning our attention to what is going on both inside and outside a brain cell, we also served the purpose of laying a foundation for the purpose of coming to a better contextual understanding of the multiple ways something could go wrong with the way a brain cell is intended to work, which, in turn, would later help us apply the legal notion of proximate cause as it relates to the death of a neuron.

"The cause, or more likely causes, of the death of a brain cell was then likened to a crime scene, a place where it could be assessed as to who or what has access or motive and whether there are accomplices or something acted as a lone wolf.

"This theory ties in well with modern research suggesting that 'we need to rethink the way we look at brain metabolism... Understanding the precise and biological mechanisms of the brain is a critical first step in disease-based research. Any misconception about biological functions—such as metabolism—will ultimately impact how scientists form hypotheses and analyze their findings. If we are looking in the wrong place, we won't be able to find the right answers.' (Citation, Maiken Nidergaard, M.D., D.M.Sc., Co-director, University of Rochester Center for Translational Neuro-Medicine, *Understanding How Nerve Cells in the Brain Produce Energy Required to Function*, News-Medical.net, 2015, Emphasis added).

"Under the heading of 'looking in the wrong place,' it was then found that there is emerging research that strongly suggests that other parts of our anatomy, other than what is just going on in the brain, should be subpoenaed and brought in for questioning for suspicion of conspiring with malice aforethought to cause Parkinson's disease.

"Indeed, as an example, it was shown there is mounting evidence of 'a major link between gut microbes and PD.' (Michael S. Okun, M.D., *Gut Bacteria and H. pylori*, Parkinson Report, National Parkinson Foundation, Spring, 2017).

"Before delving too deeply into the multiple causes as to why brain cells might be dying, in effect causing Parkinson's, an off ramp was temporarily taken to make certain no one was suffering from a fear, a prejudice, or an addiction that might be getting in the way of coming to an understanding of how critically important it is to strategically align ourselves with diet and exercise.

"The evidence did this by showing the paralyzing effect fear, prejudice, or an addiction has on our lives in a larger social context so as to drive home the point of how terribly wrong things can go when we allow these obstacles to determine our fate.

"In defense of fear, it was shown fear was actually needed by our Distant Nomadic Ancestors (DNA) for acting quickly in order to survive existential threats mostly having to do with predators with long pointy teeth, sharp claws, or poisonous fangs.

"But somewhere along the evolutionary trail, even when waning survival threats did not need to invoke the same type of response, fear, as we understood it in prehistoric days, did not evolve into a higher state of consciousness, but, instead, remained steadfast as an instinctual reaction to a new kind of fear.

"When pressed by the Court to distinguish between prehistoric fear and modern day fear, it was offered as evidence that one difference is that the threat triggering the fear, relied upon by our DNA for their survival, had a definite beginning and a definite end.

"Whereas, our more modern day fabricated fear could be likened to common everyday worrying which once set in motion has no clear endgame until we come to understand that most of what we spent so much of our lives worrying about never happens and when it does happen we have been given the tools to deal with it.

"Modern fear has the potential to keep the fearful in a perpetual state of anxiety and will continue to do so as long as the engine driving that particular type of fear is held captive by an overly active imagination deeply rooted in a dark cavern in the brain.

"The evidence showed, therefore, that we cannot enjoy the beauty unfolding before us each day if we live our lives in the hologram of a future fear.

"It was also shown by the evidence that this illogical juxtaposition of perception being fueled by misguided fear could be argued to be capable of leading to tragic consequences not only on a personal level but on a larger social level as well.

"For example, I was able to show using clear and convincing evidence that when a nation initiates a major foreign policy decision while caught in a web of fear and anger, it could easily be shown that a nation risks being diagnosed with the same mental disorder an individual would suffer if held to the same psychological standards. (Reference, *Diagnostic and Statistical Manual of Mental Disorders* (DSM-5), Fifth Edition, 2013, American Psychiatric Association.)

"For the record, the criteria triggered by fear for having suffered a diagnosis of an antisocial personality disorder included: unlawful behavior, deceitfulness, impulsivity, irritability, and aggressiveness; reckless disregard for the safety of self or others; irresponsibility; and a lack of remorse.

"So the evidence clearly shows, whether fear bullies itself to the forefront of our collective consciousness as a nation and makes us do things we otherwise would not do under normal circumstances or whether fear bullies itself to the forefront of our consciousness when we are diagnosed with Parkinson's and makes us not do things we should do, in either instance, it usually does not end as well as it otherwise could.

"Similarly, it was shown how prejudice against diet and exercise is remarkably similar to the way most other prejudices play out, which in the final analysis ends up hurting the person harboring the prejudice as much as or more than the target of the loathing.

"If left unchecked, no matter the prejudice, it risks metastasizing to the point where it becomes an all consuming creature unto itself, often to the point where the person who spawned the prejudice no longer harbors the prejudice as much as the prejudice harbors the person.

"The issue then becomes whether a person who is experiencing the depth of such despair is suffering from Post Traumatic Tribal Disorder (PTTD), i.e., the inability of a person to disassociate from an extreme ancestral prejudice.

"In that case, the best solution, as evidenced by Erwin Wilson's request for forgiveness from John Lewis for his past mistakes, was to find a way to be able to think from the orbitofrontal cortex. This is the part of the brain where a person can honestly think about the consequences of his or her actions.

"Turning our attention back to Parkinson's, it was shown that the biggest danger of a person harboring a deep-seated resentment toward exercise may, indeed, be that a person may be excluding from his or her treatment repertoire the only thing that has a remote chance of keeping brain cells alive by aerobically inducing electrochemical reactions in the brain.

"When the Court asked how to identify someone who has a prejudice against exercise, it was suggested that a litmus test would be whether or not exercise is seen as a necessary evil rather than a necessary blessing. Some people who think exercise is bad may be able to point to a specific personal experience from their past that triggered a negative neurological association that was burned into their subconscious.

"And the antidote to relieving this particular prejudice would begin by moving thought to the rational part of the brain in order to deliberate on matters related to whether the obstacle has outlived its shelf life, especially if it can be determined that the utilitarian benefits of keeping brain cells alive outweigh the prejudicial effect of bad memories associated with exercise.

"Rounding out the troublesome trio of obstacles, which has the potential to cripple a person's ability to make healthy choices regarding the use of diet and exercise to stave off the progression of Parkinson's disease, was giving into the temptation of an unhealthy addiction.

"Evidence was presented showing all addictions origi-nate in an area of the brain called the *nucleus accum-bens septi*, which receives its input from yet another part of the brain referred to as the ventral tegmental area (VTA).

"It was further shown that the nucleus accumbens septi and the ventral tegmental area are part of a system most neuroscientists refer to as the endogenous reward sys-tem, located in the limbic system.

"More specifically, it was revealed the endogenous re-ward system, which includes the VTA, projects the neu-rotransmitter dopamine to a specific part of the brain thought to control our desire for pleasure, which, again, is called the nucleus accumbens septi.

"Most importantly, in helping to overcome an addiction, is knowing there are neural pathways not only going from the VTA to the nucleus accumbens septi, where addictions are thought to take root, but also neuro pathways projecting directly from the VTA to our prefrontal cortex (rational thought) and our orbitofrontal cortex (social conscience, sense of right and wrong).

"It was also alleged that there is a greater probability of getting addicted to something unhealthy when the prefrontal cortex (rational thought) and orbitofrontal cortex (moral compass) are cut off from the endogenous reward system's complex organization of checks and balances.

"In other words, it was argued, if all decisions having to do with what causes us pleasure are made under the exclusive control of the nucleus accumbens septi, resulting from being disconnected from the prefrontal cortex and/or the orbital-frontal cortex, then things will probably go haywire until a neuronal reconnection is made.

"Then, after some comic relief, it was noted that in order for brain cells to survive the trials and tribulations of daily living, what we eat has to be factored into the equation.

"To that end, it was suggested that the food we eat determines whether we feed our brain cells good glucose or bad glucose, which may determine, in the final analysis, whether they live or die.

"Shifting gears, in an attempt to show how the human brain is composed of a multitude of parts acting in concert, it was likened to a well maintained university, where each department inculcates into its overall curriculum separate and distinct fields of study, relying for its life on a constellation of highly evolved interconnected pathways amongst departments, an infrastructure, and an administration overseeing the operations of the various brain functions.

"It was then suggested that out of all the departments that were mentioned, the most important one as far as these proceedings were concerned was the Department of Movement, which included both the extrapyramidal motor programs and the pyramidal motor system.

"It was then further explained to the Court that the pyramidal motor system plans, initiates, and executes (PIE) a movement directly to the spinal cord, whereas the extrapyramidal motor programs could be thought of as highly evolved departmental subspecialties, e.g., the basal ganglia, which does not connect directly to the spinal cord and, therefore, must pass movement information through the motor cortex.

"This can result, if in good working order, in us doing unconscious things like swinging our arms freely while walking (function of the substantia nigra in the basal ganglia).

"In addition to the various university departments, in order for each brain to function efficiently, a healthy administration was factored into its overall equation, which could be thought of as being housed in the frontal lobe, which is best known for being able to calculate, calibrate, and inculcate executive decisions, making sound judgments, and organizing planning.

"And it was then further explained how the university system is efficient so long as the information between departments and administration flows freely, but problems inevitably ensue when, like in any relationship, there is a breakdown in communication and conflict is not resolved within a prescribed period of time.

"By creating an analogy of comparing how a brain works and how a university is run, I attempted to lay a foundation so it would be easier for us to understand how medications not only help control Parkinson's symptoms, but how they can cause side effects as well.

"Even though the discovery of drugs to stop the movement disorders caused by this disease was the result of some amazing science, this discovery was tempered by the fact that, as of now, there is no known drug for this disease that can help keep brain cells alive or fix their structure so they can keep working well.

"This led to another finding that drug dosage to curb symptoms must escalate commensurate with the number of brain cells dying, and that decrease in the number of neurons depends upon the individual and what actions he or she is taking to help keep symptoms from getting out of control.

"In response to the Court's request for the names of synthetic brain drugs being marketed to curb said Parkinson's symptoms, two of the most popular medications that have been manufactured to date were offered into evidence: (1) dopamine agonists, which claim to replicate dopamine, and (2) levodopa, which claims to synthetically be able to propagate itself into actual dopamine by absorbing itself into the brain cell.

"It was further explained that the purpose of a dopamine agonist is to mimic what the neurotransmitter dopamine does by inputting movement information with an appropriate postsynaptic receptor, which, it was argued, can be a daunting task since, of the trillions of postsynaptic receptors in the brain, successful input assumes the drug is able to hook up correctly with the correct receptor on the receiving end of another brain cell, which in and of itself is pretty amazing.

"Again, no small feat since, in addition to there being trillions of receptors, I would think, it must somehow be able to know how to match excitatory sensitive keys (neurotransmitters) with excitatory sensitive locks (dendrites) and, by the same token, somehow also intuit that inhibitory sensitive keys (neurotransmitters), likewise, only fit into inhibitory sensitive locks (dendrites).

"Circling back, it was explained, levodopa was actually the first medication proven effective for treating a chronic degenerative neurologic disease, being absorbed into the bloodstream from the small intestines and traveling through the blood to the brain, where it was alleged to be converted into the active neurotransmitter dopamine. (Citation, *Parkinson's Disease: Medications,* 4th Edition, National Parkinson Foundation, 2011, p.8.)

"It was shown then that levodopa gets its religion by claiming to be able to convert itself into the real stuff, but, as pointed out, like other contraindicated, anti-evolutionary panaceas too good to be true, it was soon discovered levodopa had a tendency to lose its effectiveness at controlling symptoms of the disease in tandem with how many brain cells were dying, thus resulting, again, in a person having to take higher doses of the drug to compensate for this exponential neuronal attrition rate.

"Looking at the science through the lens of a lawyer, I humbly submitted to the Court that the manner in which brain cells die in one person, which can lead to a diagnosis of Parkinson's, may be dying for a completely different reason in another, and therefore, since each person's Parkinson's is different, the jury is still out on the issue as to whether there may be a different proximate cause(s) as to why brain cells are dying in one person in one way and dying in a wholly different way in another.

"Causation, it was argued, as it relates to Parkinson's disease, is best understood in the context that the disease is triggered when a threshold number of brain cells die in an area of the basal ganglia (substantia nigra), resulting in molecular information having difficulty passing from brain cell to brain cell, which results in making movement more difficult.

"The objective, then, was coming to a better understanding of the multiple ways in which brain cells can die, which may be the result of the particular vulnerability of the neurons in a respective person, which makes exercising control over what we have ultimate power over, diet and exercise, all the more important.

"With that said, it was then easier to understand how science has evolved, until recently, almost exclusively treating the disease with a medication targeting method model that brings something outside the brain into the brain, which, as was shown, is designed to find its way across the blood brain barrier.

"The science, arguably, again, until recently, has not made a big deal about our doing something outside the brain like aerobic exercise to cause a daily deep brain stimulation of sorts as a way of giving at risk brain cells a fighting chance to restore their structural integrity in order to stay alive because, quite frankly, the value of aerobic exercise was not always considered a valuable tool in keeping brain cells alive.

"Interesting, the evidence showed that Dr. James Parkinson, after having discovered the disease that bore his name, thought the external medicines of his era to fight the disease were scarcely warranted, and, I should add, since health clubs were not yet in vogue three hundred years ago, he apparently was unaware of the benefits of aerobic exercise, to say nothing of the powerful effect a healthy diet has in helping to keep brain cells alive.

"The Court, however, was reminded that at that time, without the benefit of the science that led to the discovery that each brain cell is a separate structural unit, let alone knowing each neuron came custom made with its own power station (mitochondria), it would have been a challenge for Dr. Parkinson to be able to connect the dots between aerobic exercise and diet and the part they play in helping to be able to maintain a healthy brain.

"With that in mind, fast forward, calling upon some of the most learned medical scholars of our day, the following brain related benefits of exercise were offered as evidence: including recent studies suggesting that exercise may have a disease-modifying effect on helping remaining dopamine cells function more efficiently; another finding showed how exercise boosts blood flow to the brain, which helps supply oxygen, glucose, and nutrients and takes away toxic substances... adding, if the deep areas of the brain are starved of healthy blood flow, there will be problems with coordination and processing complex thoughts; it was also suggested by yet another scholar that the dopamine-producing system in the substantia nigra had been better preserved in the animals that exercised; and, by yet another, exercise doesn't selectively influence anything—it adjusts the chemistry of the entire brain to restore normal signaling.

"When these two latter findings were joined together, i.e., '...the dopamine-producing system in the substantia nigra had been better preserved in the animals that exercised' (Doidge, p. 83) and '...exercise... adjusts the chemistry of the entire brain to restore normal signaling.' (Ratey, p. 135), it was argued that such findings gave credence to the integrity of the argument being made regarding the relationship between exercise and overall brain health, which has implications that go far beyond Parkinson's disease.

"Another important part of these proceedings was when it was said that our condition can get worse when brain receptors linked to Parkinson's-affected body parts are damaged to the point where they can't get clear signals to start a chemical reaction because the affected body parts aren't moving the way they normally do to do so.

"And it was emphasized that when those evolutionary motion detectors, i.e., receptors in the brain, linked to those particular motionless body parts, are not stimulated for a certain period of time, the brain cells to which they are connected may be at risk because of the reality of the phrase 'use it or lose it'.

"By way of helping to illustrate my point, what I believe happens when a person with Parkinson's uses an elliptical machine is that he or she is forcing the issue of creating a chemical reaction in the part of the brain connected to the parts of the body most affected by the disease (arms and legs), parts that might otherwise remain dormant but for the deliberate act of orchestrating movement caused by the proper use of my own aerobic exercise machine of choice.

"Deliberate aerobic movement on our part of these particular body parts affected by Parkinson's, I have to believe, might still be capable of sending signals to the applicable neuroreceptors in the part of the brain most affected by the disease, which, in turn, may cause the body to move as best it can.

"So assuming this allegation is understood and will be acted upon to the best of our ability, these proceedings will end as they began. With the now proven allegation, we each have within our control the freedom to premeditate, deliberate, and act upon movement in such a manner as to cause a chemical reaction in our brain, the intent of which is to keep brain cells alive so we might continue to be a body in motion for as long as we all shall live."

"SO HELP YOU GOD, COUNSEL?"

"SO HELP ME GOD, your Honor, and with this I rest my case."

EPILOGUE
BULLET POINTS

I SWEAR under penalty of perjury, to the best of my knowledge, that by having understood, accepted, and acted upon the following fundamental truths, which I believe to be factual, an appreciable amount of my mental and physical health has been restored after having been diagnosed with Parkinson's disease nearly ten years ago.

NUMBER ONE: Going back in time, it is important to know our Distant Nomadic Ancestors (DNA) greatly relied upon the parts of their brain that control movement in order to overcome imminent threats to life and limb posed by prehistoric predators.

. . .

NUMBER TWO: For me, I felt a connection between how our DNA used movement to avert such an existential threat and how we with Parkinson's might also use movement to tame what can clearly be thought of as a new age predator.

NUMBER THREE: By weaving together these two threads of time, with minor alterations, it made it easier for me to understand how in both eras there was a critical need to awaken certain neurons in the brain that control movement in order to survive.

NUMBER FOUR: Averting threats, whether posed by a prehistoric predator or those inherent in having Parkinson's disease, I found it helpful to know that legs and limbs, essential in both circumstances, are directly connected to a specific part of the brain responsible for the mediation of certain motor movements.

NUMBER FIVE: It is important to know that in prehistoric times, we relied on yet another part of the brain (amygdala), which controls the appropriate fight or flight response, in order to set in motion the necessary neuro-chemical reaction that helped us navigate past an immediate existential threat.

NUMBER SIX: In more modern times, in order to tame the beast burdening us, we are now better off not responding so much from our fear center, where we are expected to fight or take flight, but from yet another part of the brain (the frontal lobe) in order, instead, to calculate the most rational response in order to tame the beast within.

NUMBER SEVEN: So, then, rather than creating the false perception we must fight with or flee from Parkinson's, we, instead, need to use another part of the brain (the frontal lobe), which will reveal to us the advantages of figuring out a way to live a healthy life by, instead, counterintuitively, domesticating the disease.

NUMBER EIGHT: As it relates to coping with a progressive brain disease, strategically, we have come to the point in our history where it may make more sense to rely on the part of the brain (the frontal lobe) that has evolved for the purposes of fostering motivation, emotional control, good judgment, skillful problem solving, and decision making.

. . .

NUMBER NINE: In other words, the futility of attempting to tame Parkinson's from the vantage point of the competing area of the brain, which has evolved primarily for purposes of reacting to an immediate threat, becomes more and more obvious when the disease seems to thrive in a cerebral environment that relies mostly upon fear or anger as a means of responding to an existing problem. (Parenthetically, which probably also explains why history seems to have a knack for repeating itself.)

NUMBER TEN: Even with that said, some people diagnosed with Parkinson's will still begin the healing process by thinking they can 'fight' an undefeatable foe, and when they fail to achieve a desired outcome, what will become remarkably predictable is the temptation they have to take 'flight' from the agony of defeat by seeking a quick retreat into the world of either drugs or alcohol.

NUMBER ELEVEN: Successful domestication of the beast, on the other hand, will be found by most to be a more viable alternative when done from the vantage point of the rational brain, assuming a person can negotiate his or her way to the frontal lobe without being waylaid by such impediments as future fear, prejudice against exercise, or succumbing to an addiction.

NUMBER TWELVE: Taming, rather than fighting, Parkinson's might be found to be especially uncomplicated by those who have recently been diagnosed, especially if they have the requisite discipline and motivation to act in their own best interest from the very moment of their diagnosis.

NUMBER THIRTEEN: Taking action begins by building a foundation for the safe construction of an imaginary three legged stool supported by aerobic exercise, the consumption of only good foods for the brain, and a reasonable medical regimen, any part of which, if missing, will, more likely than not, sabotage the process of restoring vitality to dying brain cells, which is clearly our main objective.

NUMBER FOURTEEN: Paradoxically, again, becoming aware we each have under our control the ability to start the process of domesticating the disease by simply igniting a chemical reaction in the brain by exercising in a certain way will not be enough incentive for most to take any meaningful action until they have a clearer picture of the neurological firestorm they each have the power to create.

NUMBER FIFTEEN: With that in mind, biologically speaking, when we cause legs and limbs to move repetitively for a prolonged period, ideally on an elliptical machine, a part of the brain to which these appendages are connected (substantia nigra) allows brain cells to react by causing synaptic vesicles containing the neurotransmitter dopamine to fuse with a brain cell's presynaptic membrane, causing dopamine to be released into a synapse, freeing the chemical to interact with receptors (dendrites) on another brain cell, which exists for the sole purpose of replicating the same chemical reaction, which is all just a fancy way of saying that fluid motion should be restored to a certain degree each time we trigger this particular chemical reaction by meaningfully exercising aerobically.

NUMBER SIXTEEN: Domesticating the disease, then, begins by allowing the rational part of our brain to trumpet a clarion call to arms (and legs) to move harmoniously for an extended period of time each day, in order to electrochemically excite brain cells in a certain part of the brain to the point whereby they somehow each sense, as has been the case throughout time, that they have been naturally selected to play a critical role in the guarantee of our survival, that is, if we are willing to play our part in allowing them to fulfill their destiny.

RESOURCES

"It bears repeating that Parkinson's disease really is not the disease of your parents anymore where you just take medication and wait for bad things to happen. Rather, it is possible to change this disease by using a specific set of powerful tools to keep brain cells alive.

"While you can rely on modern medicine to treat the symptoms, it is your personal responsibility to make sure you improve the structural integrity of each brain cell to keep it alive. It is time for you to go past treating the symptoms and move on to treating the disease by flooding the brain with blood, oxygen, and good glucose. This is the key everyone has been looking for.

"I challenge you to set aside your casual treatment of diet and exercise as support. You must really hit home for yourself the importance of both diet and exercise for keeping brain cells alive. You must take on the responsibility to do that on your own, realizing how important both are for keeping brain cells alive."

Jerry Hurtubise, J.D.

RESOURCE LIST

Amen, D.G. (2008). Magnificent Mind at Any Age. New York: Harmony Books.

Bachman, R. (2015, July 6). Treadmills Unplugged: A Gym Workout Powered by Your Feet. The Wall Street Journal. https://www.wsj.com/articles/treadmills-un plugged-a-gym-workout-powered-by-your-feet-1436202306

Berger, A. (2017). The Alzheimer's Antidote. White River Junction: Chelsea Green Publishing.

Bishop, R. (2018, June 7). Leg Exercise is Critical to Brain and Nervous System Health. Frontiers in Neuroscience. https://blog.frontiersin.org/2018/06/07/neuro science-leg-exercise-brain-nervous-system-health/

Dalloway, T.P. (2011). Training Your Brain for Dummies (p.158). West Sussex: A. John Wiley and Sons, Ltd. Publication.

Diagnostic and Statistical Manual of Mental Disorders (DSM-5), Fifth Edition. (2013) American Psychiatric Association.

Doidge, N. (2015). The Brain's Way of Healing. New York: Viking Press.

Fernandes, J. (2017, January). Aberrant Astrocytes May Lead to Parkinson's, Other Neurodegenerative Diseases. https://parkinsonsnewstoday.com/news/aberrant-astrocytes-may-lead-parkinsons-other-neurodegenerative-diseases/

Fitzgerald, S. (2018, January 25). Early PD Patients May Benefit from Exercising at a High Intensity. Neurology Today. https://journals.lww.com/neurotodayonline/toc/2018/01250

Kohgaku, E. et al. (2017, June 21). Wild-type monomeric a-synuclein can impair vesicle endocytosis and synaptic fidelity via tubulin polymerization at the calyx of Held. Journal of Neuroscience. https://pubmed.ncbi.nlm.nih.gov/28576942/

Liddell, S.A. et al. (2017, January). Neurotoxic Reactive Astrocytes Are Induced by Activated Microglia. Nature. https://www.nature.com/articles/nature21029

Martinez, M.E. (2013). Future Bright, A Transforming Vision of Human Intelligence. New York Oxford University Press.

National Institute of Health. (2013). NIH Publication No. 13-7907 (p. 2). https://www.nih.gov/about-nih/nih-publications-list

National Institute of Neurological Disorders and Stroke. (2013, September, NIH Publication No. 13-2252). The Dementias. https://www.ninds.nih.gov/

National Parkinson Foundation. (2011). Parkinson's Disease: Medications, 4th Edition. https://www.parkinson.org/

National Priorities Project. https://www.nationalpriorities.org/cost-of/

Nidergaard, M. (2015). Understanding How Nerve Cells in the Brain Produce Energy Required to Function. https://www.news-medical.net/news/20150425/Understanding-how-nerve-cells-in-the-brain-produce-energy-required-to-function.aspx

Okun, M.S. (2017, Spring). Gut Bacteria and H.pylori. Parkinson Report, National Parkinson Foundation. https://www.parkinson.org/

Paddock, C. (2017, June 21). Autoimmunity May Have Role in Parkinson's Disease. Medical News Today. https://www.medicalnewstoday.com/articles/318029

Parashos, A. (2013). Navigating Life with Parkinson Disease (p.191). New York: Oxford University.

Parkinson, J. (1817). Essay on the Shaking Palsy (p.62). London: Whittingham and Rowland.

Perier, C., Vila, M. (2012, February). Mitochondrial Biology and Parkinson's Disease. Cold Spring Harbor Perspectives in Medicine. https://pubmed.ncbi.nlm.nih.gov/22355801/

Ratey, J.J. (2008), Spark, The Revolutionary New Science of Exercise and the Brain. New York: Little Brown and Company.

Reynolds, G. (2017, December 13). Exercise May Aid Parkinson's Disease, but Make It Intense. The New York Times. https://www.nytimes.com/2017/12/13/well/move/exercise-may-aid-parkinsons-disease-but-make-it-intense.html

Turnbull, D. (2013, January). Powering the Brain: An Introduction to Mitochondria. Think Neuroscience Wordpress. https://thinkneuroscience.wordpress.com/2013/01/16/an-introduction-to-mitochondria/

Zhang, J. et al. (2018, January). Mitochondrial Function and Autophagy: Integrating Proteotoxic, Redox, and Metabolic Stress in Parkinson's Disease. Journal of Neurochemistry. https://onlinelibrary.wiley.com/doi/10.1111/jnc.14308

ACKNOWLEDGMENTS

My wife and care partner extraordinaire, Catherine, who with every fiber of her being has created for me a well of living water, the depth of which can only be measured in the amount of joy she shares with me at the dawn of each new day.

My son Peter, who for as long as I can remember, has been an inspiration to me in the way he lives his life, the source of which can only be understood in the context of being something truly divine.

My sister, Mary Ann, without reservation I can say, but for her dedication to this project, my book would never have seen the light of day, left, instead, to languish amongst the thousands and thousands of other more deserving manuscripts, whose fate would probably have been much different had they had the relentless perseverance of a loyal sister on their side.

The pack at Winterwolf Press, Laura, Christine, Jeffrey, Jeanette, Claire, Jose, Aubrie, and Russ who, like so many angels who just seem to magically appear in my life at exactly the right moment, generously have shared their skills to turn an ordinary writer like myself into an extraordinary writer.

My movement disorder neurologist at UCSF, Chad Christine, M.D., has always been far ahead of the neurological curve in singing the praises of using aerobic exercise as a way of slowing down the progression of Parkinson's disease.

My online fitness gurus, Lisa and SteF at PD-Connect, whose daily exercise classes make me stronger, more balanced, with better posture, and keep me less fearful of moving forward in my life physically and emotionally, all in all making it my second favorite hour each day.

My law partner of nearly 30 years, Greg Winslow, who for all that time carried me on his formidable coattails so we together, could evolve to a point where we could reliably be trusted to represent in a court of law those who suffered a traumatic brain injury.

ABOUT THE AUTHOR

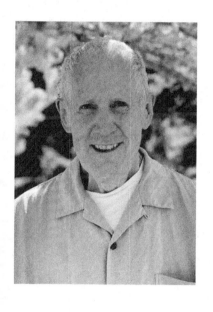

A seasoned San Francisco trial attorney, Jerry Hurtubise was diagnosed with Parkinson's Disease and embarked on a quest to utilize his extensive knowledge from litigating head trauma cases to explore effective methods for managing his disease. Determined to live a fulfilling life alongside his beloved wife, Catherine, of thirty-five years, Jerry's journey led him to identify the crucial role of vigorous aerobic exercise and a brain-healthy diet in mitigating the effects of Parkinson's.

His book, "Parkinsonian Democracy," is set in the imaginative space of the United States District Court of Public Opinion where Hurtubise conveys through the voice of the seasoned trial attorney character, Christian Cultura, compelling evidence for the critical impact of exercise and nutrition on slowing the progress of Parkinson's disease.

With a rich understanding of the human condition and its evolution and the support of irrefutable scientific evidence, Hurtubise argues for a shift in our thinking, emphasizing the need to engage the rational parts of the brain rather than persist in modes of thought that may no longer serve us. He knows how many diagnosed can keep their focus on the progressive degeneration of Parkinson's and become overwhelmed and trapped in the belief that their ability to maintain wellness is out of their control.

Jerry Hurtubise invites those diagnosed with Parkinson's to find refuge in a "Parkinsonian Democracy." Until there is a cure, "Parkinsonian Democracy" offers a fresh perspective and a call to action for those battling Parkinson's, bringing a ray of hope into the lives of those in need.

Jerry Hurtubise, J.D.

State Bar of California (1980-Present)

San Francisco City Attorney (1980-1984)

Civil Practice,
Including Brain Injury Litigation (1985-2013)

Editor, Citizens Alert of Chicago (1976-1977)

Community Organizer,
United Farm Workers (1975-1976)

Author, *The Spiritual Apprenticeship of a Curious Catholic* (ACTA, 2005)

"...these beautifully written memoirs of a Catholic as a
young man could not have come
at a more opportune time."
—Theodore Hesburgh, University of Notre Dame

"Occasionally something is written causing us to reflect
upon and more fully appreciate our common Catholic
experience. This refreshingly unmoralistic, often poetic,
book is one such experience."
—Helen Prejean

"...shows a great sensitivity to words, and even more important, shows a great sensitivity to life, and shares both
skills with us in an enriching way."
—Senator Paul Simon

Jesuit Honor Society (1975)

San Francisco Bar Association Award (2011)

University of San Francisco School of Law J.D. (1980)

Medill School of Journalism, Northwestern University (Summer 1975)

Loyola University of Chicago, History B.A. (1975)

Marian High School of Mishawaka, Indiana (1971)

ALSO BY WINTERWOLF PRESS

If you enjoyed "Parkinsonian Democracy: A Legal Fiction Advocacy for Diet & Exercise for Parkinson's" you will also love these additional Winterwolf Press titles.

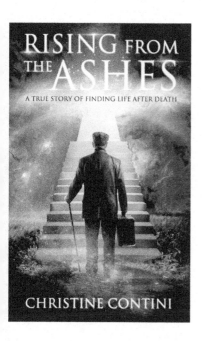

CHRISTINE CONTINI

Author of Rising From the Ashes, A True Story of Finding Life After Death

In this intriguing narrative, Contini awakens her latent abilities to interact with her now-deceased Uncle Ricky, aiding him in his journey to cross over. Her experiences challenge conventional spiritual beliefs and provide illuminating insights into the death and dying process.

The book dives into a range of essential themes, examining how grief can tether the dead to the earthly realm, and introducing the concept of the "Angle of Acceleration," a novel understanding of the mechanics that enable the transition of the soul to the other side. Contini further explores the implications of cremation at the soul level, offering a fresh perspective on this ancient practice.

The wealth of information presented in this engrossing short story shows that the process of dying is not an isolated experience exclusive to the deceased, but rather, a communal endeavor involving both the living and the dead.

You are invited to accompany Contini on her extraordinary journey, gaining a deeper understanding of life, death, and the intriguing spaces in between.

CHRISTINE CONTINI

Author of Death: Awakening to Life, Seeds Planted

This heartfelt and compassionate collection of adventures dares to awaken the reader to the amazing truth of what lies after death and shows the awe-inspiring beginnings that can be birthed from what many think of as the end.

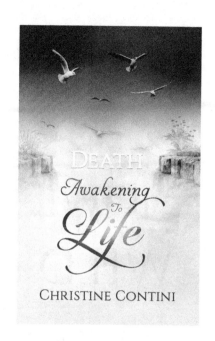

At the young age of 37, Christine Contini experienced a sudden cardiac death. Over 40 minutes later, she returned from the other side, carrying the keys to unlock profound understanding and seemingly supernatural abilities. Dying allowed Christine to awaken to humanity's natural energetic potentials and pierce the veil between the physical and energetic worlds.

In *Death: Awakening to Life, Seeds Planted*, Christine takes us on a journey through life, death, and rebirth. She presents fascinating information about what happens after we die and describes, from first-hand experience, the many pitfalls that can entangle the dying and their loved ones during the death process.

Christine's messages enable us to recognize that death is not the end of anything, but the return to all we know yet somehow forgot.

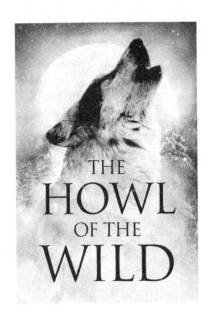

By WINTERWOLF PRESS

Howl of the Wild, A Nature Anthology

This extraordinary collection emerges from a multitude of voices – poets, creative writers, and nature enthusiasts – all drawn together by their shared reverence for the environment.

"Howl of the Wild" is more than a simple anthology; it is an artistic tapestry woven together with threads of vivid narratives, emotive poetry, and poignant reflections, all inspired by nature's splendor. Each page takes the reader on a journey into the heart of the wilderness, unravelling its mysteries and marvels.

Contributors such as Melissa Calderon-Rougié, Burton L. Carlson, Suzanne Cottrell, and Gregory Luce, among many others, lend their unique literary voices to this collection. Their words echo with a deep appreciation for the wild, resonating with the stirring call of animals, the whisper of trees, and the silent strength of mountains.

Engross yourself in the rich tapestry of "Howl of the Wild: A Nature Anthology", and journey through a kaleidoscope of sensory experiences as you delve into the untamed beauty of our natural world.

FOR MORE TITLES AND ANNOUNCEMENTS BY WINTERWOLF PRESS, FOLLOW THE WOLF CODE

Interested in joining the Winterwolf Pack?

Check to see the current submission status.

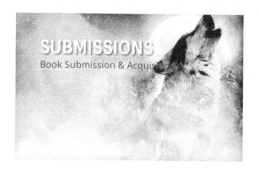

Made in the USA
Monee, IL
11 January 2024

51594933R00164